# PAIN-FREE PERIODS

Looks at the causes of difficult menstruation and shows how
this problem can be helped by diet, exercise, stress-reducing
measures and other natural remedies, including evening
primrose oil.

# PAIN-FREE PERIODS

## Natural Ways to Overcome Menstrual Problems

*by*

## STELLA WELLER

THORSONS PUBLISHING GROUP
Wellingborough * New York

First published 1986

British Library Cataloguing in Publication Data

Weller, Stella
  Pain-free periods: natural ways to
    overcome menstrual problems
  1. Dysmenorrhea   2. Naturopathy
  I. Title
  618.1'72      RG181

  ISBN 0-7225-1195-7

Printed and bound in Great Britain by
Richard Clay (The Chaucer Press) Ltd,
Bungay, Suffolk

# Contents

# Introduction

Every month thousands of women all over the world suffer from *dysmenorrhoea,* or difficult menstrual periods. The cost to industry, in terms of lowered productivity, is very high indeed. Many women show symptoms and are not feeling or functioning optimally for two to three months out of each year. This translates into millions of pounds, dollars and marks, representing between three and eight per cent of the total wage bill. The price paid in respect of human resources is not so readily calculated, however. For who can place monetary value on human distress and pain and suffering?

For many years, I have lived and worked closely with hundreds of women. I know for a fact the agony that many of them experience at that certain time each month when the menstrual period becomes an unwelcome reality. Many of my nursing colleagues in England called it 'the curse'. On one gynaecology ward where I worked, the Sister in charge would compassionately excuse us from duty for a couple of hours' respite from the nagging menstrual cramps that prevented us from carrying out our duties effectively.

When I worked in the Caribbean as an airline steward-ess—again in close collaboration with dozens of women—I watched some of my co-workers struggle to keep a smile on their faces, while serving passengers in flight, simultaneously bearing the pain of dysmenorrhoea. One of them became nauseous and almost fainted on two occasions that I worked with her, because of excruciating pain. She told me that when she worked as a cashier at a well-known bank, she invariably took to her bed for two days in each month to recover from the distress of nausea, pain and vomiting which accompanied her menstrual periods. I could relate many more similar anecdotes that confirm how disabling dysmenorrhoea is to innumerable women, and how adversely it affects those who employ them.

There are other repercussions also. People who live and work with those experiencing painful menstruation suffer as well. This is because the condition is often preceded or accompanied by symptoms ranging from mild irritability to deep depression, and a host of others, collectively referred to as the Premenstrual Syndrome, or PMS. Husbands, boyfriends, children, parents and co-workers are not infrequently unhappily affected. In fact, the depression accompanying or preceding dysmenorrhoea can be so severe as to drive the sufferer to crime!

One such case involved a thirty-year-old woman in England. She stabbed a barmaid to death. The doctor who visited her in prison diagnosed her as suffering from PMS at the time of misdeed.

Another case, also in England, was of a thirty-seven-year-old woman who had quarrelled with her lover. In a frenzy, she drove her car at him and killed him. At her court trial she pleaded guilty of manslaughter, on grounds of 'diminished responsibility'. The plea was accepted after consideration of reports by a physician and two psychiatrists. At the time of the offence, this woman had been experiencing the debilitating symptoms associated with menstruation. They were aggravated by her lover's provocation and contributed to her state of 'diminished responsibility'. This is the second occasion on which the British courts have accepted PMS as a disease of the mind. In France, PMS is recognized as a cause of temporary insanity or incompetence in some women.

We now know that mind and body are very intimately linked, and that changes in the latter inevitably affect the former. During the few days before the menstrual blood flow, when complex chemical changes are taking place in the body, concentration, co-ordination and mood can be affected. Evidence for this is seen in the number of on-the-job accidents that take place, the number of complaints made about bad-tempered service, saleswomen and receptionists, and the poor performance at examinations by young women who are usually very bright.

This book throws light on the many contributing causes of menstrual difficulty—a truly multi-dimensional problem with physical and psychological components—and offers safe, effective and natural ways of dealing with each of these causes. The beauty of the treatments suggested and described in detail is that they produce no unpleasant or destructive side-effects, as do hormonal treatments and other methods involving drugs or surgery. They have, as well, the advantage of promoting overall health and of inspiring life-enhancing attitudes. Above all, they help to give a certain sense of control over one's life—an issue of increasing importance to women.

I do hope that you will persevere in applying several of the suggestions that I have outlined, and that you will reap the benefits their faithful application can bring—the experience of pain-free menstrual periods.

# CHAPTER 1

# A Look at the Pelvis

Since several of the structures involved in menstruation ('periods') lie within the pelvis, let's take a look at that part of the female anatomy.

Your pelvis, or pelvic girdle, lies between your upper body and your legs. It consists of the *sacrum,* the *coccyx* and two *innominate* (hip) *bones*.

The *sacrum* is a triangular bone situated at the lower end of the vertebral column (spine). It is wedged between the two innominate bones and forms the back of the pelvic cavity.

The *coccyx* ('tail bone') consists of four or five rudimentary vertebrae (bones that make up the spine), fused into one. It lies below the sacrum and articulates, or connects, with it to form a joint.

The two *innominate bones* (or 'nameless' bones) are located one on each side of the pelvis and unite in front at the *symphysis pubis* (the bony eminence under the pubic hair). The innominate bones are flat and irregularly shaped; they are formed by the union of three bones that unite at the acetabulum, a cup-shaped cavity on the external surface which receives the head of each femur (thigh bone) to form hip joints. The bones uniting to form an innominate bone are the *ilium* (you can sometimes feel its crest at the front of the hip), the *pubis* and the *ischium* ('sitting bone').

The bony pelvis is divided into the *true pelvis*, or pelvic basin, which is the lower part, and the false pelvis, which is formed by the upper portion of the iliac bones (referring to the ilium). The true pelvis is the bony basin formed by the ischium and pubis, which make up the sides and front, and the sacrum and coccyx at the back. The brim of the pelvis is formed by the promontory (projecting part) of the sacrum at the back, and crest of the pubis at the front. These form the rim or basin-like upper margin of the bony cavity.

It is interesting to note that the female pelvis differs from the male pelvis in that it is wider and shallower. The pelvic inlet is larger and more circular than that of the male; the ischial tuberosities ('sitting bones') are farther apart and the coccyx is more movable.

The joints of the pelvis are as follows:

*The sacro-iliac* joints are where the sacrum connects on each side with the articular surfaces of the ilium. Because very strong ligaments unite these joints, movement is limited.

The *symphysis pubis* is where the pubic bones join in front. They are composed of cartilage and are separated by a pad of the same material. This is a partially movable joint.

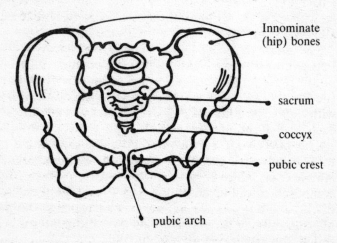

Fig. 1
Drawing of the female pelvis

## The Pelvic Floor

The structures lying within the boundaries of the pelvic outlet form the floor of the pelvis, or the pelvic floor.

Two sets of muscles, the *levator ani* muscles, or levatores ani, and the *coccygeus* form what is known as the *pelvic diaphragm* (in contrast with the respiratory diaphragm involved in the breathing process).

The *perineum*, which is part of the pelvic floor, is the lowest part of the torso, or trunk. It is divided into an anterior (front) area (urogenital area), a posterior (anal) area and a central part called the *perineal body*. This is strong, fibrous, muscular tissue lying between the vaginal opening and the rectum (back passage). It may be torn during childbirth.

## Contents of the Pelvis

The *urinary bladder* is located directly behind the symphysis pubis, and the rectum lies at the back of the pelvic cavity, following the curve of the sacrum.

Lymphatic vessels and glands, nerve and blood vessels all lie within the pelvis. Also located in the pelvis are the uterus and its ligaments, and the uterine tubes and ovaries.

The *uterus* is a thick, muscular, pear-shaped organ lying between the rectum (behind) and the bladder (in front). Its body (fundus) tips forward toward the bladder. Its cervix (neck), which is the narrower part, communicates below with the vagina. Ligaments, ovaries and uterine tubes lie on each side of the uterus.

The outer coat of the uterus, which covers the upper three-quarters of the organ, is called the *peritoneum*. The middle coat, which forms the main structure of the organ, is composed of plain, unstriped muscle and a special type of tissue called *areolar tissue*, such as that which surrounds the breast nipples in the female. This layer of the uterus is richly supplied with blood and lymphatic vessels and nerves. The inner lining of the uterus, which is composed of mucous membrane (so called because it secretes mucus), is known as the *endometrium*.

## The Supports of the Uterus

The supports of the uterus are as follows:

The *levatores ani* (or levator ani muscles), which form the floor of the pelvis, support the rectum and aid defecation (bowel movement).

The *utero-sacral* ligaments pass from the uterus to the sacrum.

The *transverse ligaments* pass from the cervix (neck) of the uterus to the side walls of the pelvis and help keep the uterus in mid-line.

There are also the *broad ligaments*, two wide folds of peritoneum, which pass from the sides of the uterus and are richly supplied with blood vessels lying within their folds.

The *round ligaments* pass from the sides of the uterus, just below and in front of the entrance of the fallopian tubes. They pass through the inguinal (groin) canal, on each side, and attach to the labia majora (part of the external genitals).

## Other Structures Inside the Pelvis

Other structures within the pelvis are:

The *fallopian* (uterine) *tubes*. These pass, one on each side, from the upper part of the uterus toward the sides of the pelvis. They are about 10cm (4 inches) long, being narrower at their attachment to the uterus. The larger end has finger-like processes, one of which is attached to an ovary.

The function of the fallopian tubes is to act as a passage for ova (eggs, singular, *ovum*) travelling from the ovary to the uterus, and for sperm going from the uterus toward the ovary.

The *ovaries*. These are two almond-shaped glands located one on each side of the uterus, below the fallopian tubes. They produce ova and the hormones *oestrogen* and *progesterone*, which control menstruation. The production of these hormones is, in turn, controlled by the pituitary gland located in the brain. Oestrogens are secreted by the ovaries from childhood until after the menopause. At puberty and throughout adult life, until the menopause, an additional number of oestrogens is produced. Progesterone, also produced by the ovaries, continues the work started by the oestrogens in preparing the lining of the uterus for possible pregnancy each month. Note that *progesterone inhibits menstruation,* and that as long as its secretion persists, menstruation cannot take place.

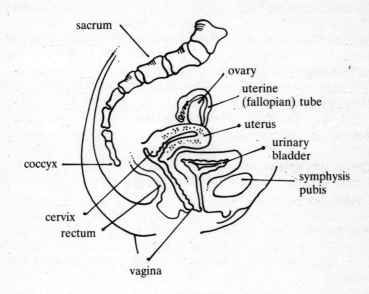

Fig. 2
Drawing of the contents of the female pelvis (side view)

## The Menstrual Cycle

The menstrual cycle prepares your body for pregnancy. If pregnancy does not occur, your body literally abandons its elaborate preparations and begins a brand-new cycle. For convenience, think of the menstrual cycle as lasting twenty-eight days (it can be as short as eighteen and as long as forty).

Several structures are intimately involved in this complex, yet superbly co-ordinated, process. They are: the hypothalamus and the pituitary gland, both located in the brain; and the ovaries, fallopian tubes and uterus, all of which are situated in the pelvis.

The *hypothalamus* (from Greek *hypo*, under, and *thalamos*, chamber) is located in the forebrain, beneath the thalamus. It appears to influence the integration, or 'assembling in orderly fashion', of emotional expression. It also exercises control of metabolic processes, such as the regulation of body temperature and endocrine gland secretion (hormones). Because of the latter, the hypothalamus plays a vital role in emotions generated by stress—one of the crucial factors involved in the pain of menstruation and its associated signs and symptoms.

With specific regard to the menstrual cycle, the hypothalamus stimulates the *pituitary gland* (an endocrine gland, about the size of a pea, located in the base of the brain) to release hormones that initiate changes in the ovaries and uterus. These changes may be grouped into four sets, or phases, for the sake of simplicity.

### The proliferative phase (phase of rapid reproduction)

— Lasts from ten to fourteen days.

— In response to a signal from the hypothalamus, the pituitary gland releases FSH (Follicle-Stimulating Hormone). FSH influences the maturation of some ova inside the ovaries. These ova become *primary follicles*. They develop a double layer of cells around them and upon maturation are known as *graafian follicles*.

— The graafian follicles begin to produce *oestrogen*, which stimulates the endometrium (lining of the uterus) to thicken in preparation for receiving a fertilized ovum. Oestrogen also facilitates the passage of the mature ovum through the fallopian tube, and changes the quality of the mucus in the cervix (neck of uterus) to make it easier for sperm to enter the uterus.

— The now-high level of oestrogen stimulates the pituitary gland to release LH (Luteinizing Hormone), which in turn stimulates ovulation. Now one of the graafian follicles travels to the edge of the ovary and takes on a blister-like appearance. When the blister bursts, the ovum is released and usually enters the corresponding fallopian tube.

It is interesting to note that, as the ovary releases an ovum, some women experience a type of pelvic pain known as *mittelschmerz* (mid-cycle pain).

### The secretory phase

— Lasts from ten to fourteen days.

—The ruptured graafian follicle transforms itself into a *corpus luteum* (yellow body) and begins to produce *progesterone*.

— The pituitary gland now secretes LTH (Luteo-Tropic Hormone) which helps the corpus luteum to develop.

— The progesterone secreted by the corpus luteum brings about further changes in the uterine lining, making it thicker (between 4 and 6mm) and softer.

It is significant that, toward the end of this phase, the body tends to retain fluid, resulting in congestion and consequent discomfort.

### The pre-menstrual phase

— Lasts one to two days.

— If the ovum does not become fertilized, the corpus luteum diminishes in size and activity.

— As the corpus luteum degenerates, oestrogen and progesterone levels drop sharply.

— The blood vessels inside the uterus contract, supplying less nourishment to the uterine lining, which then breaks down for lack of blood and oxygen. Bleeding and shedding of the lining begin. Note that the abdominal cramps, which many women experience shortly before menstrual bleeding starts, are probably due to the degeneration of the uterine lining.

## The menstrual phase

— Lasts four to five days.

— Abdominal cramps may occur during the first day or two of this phase.

— Between 60 and 180ml of fluid, containing blood cells, fragments of uterine lining and various secretions, are discharged through the vagina (passage from uterus to external genitals).

— As this phase starts, other ova begin maturing—to start a whole new menstrual cycle.

The menstrual phase overlaps the first few days of the proliferative phase.

# CHAPTER 2

# Difficult Menstruation: The Types and Causes

Difficult menstruation, or *dysmenorrhoea* as it is technically known, has traditionally been categorized as either primary or secondary.

## Secondary Dysmenorrhoea

*Secondary dysmenorrhoea* is a condition in which periods were normal to begin with but, because of some disease or other process in the pelvis, painful menstruation developed.

This type of dysmenorrhoea can be caused by pelvic infection, tumours of the uterus, narrowing of the cervix following surgical procedures, certain abnormalities present at birth, the use of an intra-uterine contraceptive device (IUD), and relaxation of uterine supports secondary to childbearing. It can also be due to a condition called endometriosis, in which fragments of endometrium (uterine lining) appear and function in places other than the uterus (e.g. the ovaries, uterine ligaments and urinary bladder).

Depending on the cause of secondary dysmenorrhoea, the signs and symptoms may first appear at a young age or, indeed, in later adulthood. For example, in some young women, the hymen (fold of membrane at the entrance of the vagina) has no opening (imperforate hymen). Menstruation occurs, but the blood cannot escape through the vagina because the hymen totally obstructs it. Monthly discomfort and pain result, and the treatment is usually surgical incision of the hymen. Difficult menstruation beginning in later adulthood may be due to pelvic inflammatory disease or one of the other causes already mentioned.

The pain of secondary dysmenorrhoea may vary from dull to sharp, depending on its cause. It may occur on one side of the body or on both sides. It may radiate to the thighs and lower back, although it may not. The first appearance of discomfort and pain may coincide with the start of the menstrual flow, but it may precede it. Often, these unpleasant symptoms last the entire period.

Depending on the specific cause of this type of menstrual difficulty, signs and symptoms may range from fever (as in pelvic infection) to heavy bleeding (as in pelvic tumours or the presence of an IUD).

The treatment for secondary dysmenorrhoea depends, of course, on the underlying cause. If you have reason to believe that your menstrual difficulties may be related to one of the foregoing causes, it is important that you see your doctor for an examination.

## Primary Dysmenorrhoea

*Primary dysmenorrhoea* usually starts within a few months after a regular pattern of menstrual cycles with ovulation is established. (In some periods, ovulation does not occur. This typically happens in the first two years of a woman's menstruating life.)

## An Historical Background to Dysmenorrhoea

In the early 1900s, primary dysmenorrhoea was thought to be caused by a 'tipped' (retroverted) uterus or a 'tight' (stenotic) cervix, and surgical correction was the treatment of choice. Other attributed causes were faulty posture, overweight and lack of exercise, and treatments were geared accordingly.

But none of the foregoing 'cures' worked. In the 1930s and 1940s, scientists began to put forth theories about hormonal imbalances, in which an excess of oestrogen or a deficiency of progesterone was the culprit implicated in dysmenorrhoea and its associated symptoms.

Pregnancy was often recommended as a solution and brought relief to many women for some years following childbirth. It was not, however, a practicable 'cure' for everyone.

Then in the 1960s, behavioural researchers sought psychological explanations for dysmenorrhoea and did indeed come up with some, including feelings of rejected womanhood and maternal conditioning. They also threw light on some negative behavioural changes associated with the menstrual cycle. Among these were:

— increased irritability, pessimism and a tendency to violence;

— decreased self-confidence and feelings of self-worth, sometimes resulting in suicide or attempted suicide; and

— decreased concentration, co-ordination and performance, leading to higher accident rates.

Using the foregoing psychological symptoms as a basis, doctors began prescribing psychotropic drugs to affect psychic function, behaviour and experience, as well as powerful narcotics. Women who had been performing their duties through a haze of pain were now doing so through a drug-induced fog. Doctors also recommended that their 'patients' drastically restrict their activities.

In treating the symptoms of dysmenorrhoea, instead of the underlying causes, doctors ignored the fact that although psychological factors do influence a person's perception of pain, they are not necessarily the cause of that pain.

When the oral contraceptive pill (the Pill) came on the market, many women who had previously experienced painful periods found that it relieved their menstrual distress. Accordingly, physicians did not hesitate to prescribe the Pill as the treatment of choice for dysmenorrhoea, although they did not fully understand what caused it. The synthetic hormones (oestrogen and progestins) that are contained in the Pill arrest ovulation and limit the growth of the uterine lining, both of which seem to contribute to menstrual discomforts.

Contributory also is the presence of chemical substances called *prostaglandins*, found in menstrual secretions. These are hormone-like substances that play a role in the functions of reproductive organs. The name derives from the prostate (male sex gland), because prostaglandins were first discovered in semen. They are present, though, in many parts of the body.

Prostaglandins are made by the uterine lining. Their quantity increases greatly before menstruation. The menstrual secretions of women who ovulate contain about five times the quantity of prostaglandins of those of non-ovulating women. In fact, women who don't ovulate hardly ever complain of dysmenorrhoea.

Prostaglandins have a very powerful effect on smooth muscle, such as that of which the uterus is composed. They cause it to contract, and it is this contraction of the uterus that seems to produce some of the pain of menstruation. (In fact, prostaglandins appear to play a part in initiating labour in pregnant women, and to increase in quantity as labour progresses.) When scientists administered prostaglandins to female subjects, uterine contractions occurred and symptoms of dysmenorrhoea appeared. These included flushing of the skin, nausea and fainting. Prostaglandins also appear to influence blood-pressure, the clumping of platelets (blood cells concerned with clotting), activity of the stomach and intestines and the release of sex hormones.

At first glance, it stands to reason that if prostaglandins produce all these unpleasant and debilitating symptoms, inhibiting their action would result in 'cure'. Clinicians therefore began to prescribe prostaglandin-inhibiting medications, such as aspirin, indomethacin (Indocin), ibuprofen (Motrin), naproxen (Naprosyn) and Mefenamic acid (Ponstel); these are medications that, according to one text, are supposedly 'relatively free of side-effects'.

These drugs, however, act upon the nervous system and are not without untoward symptoms. The side-effects of aspirin include ringing in the ears, headache, dizziness, drowsiness, thirst, sweating, stomach and intestinal upsets and bleeding. Indocin can reactivate latent infections and produce marked nervous system manifestations. Ponstel may produce nervous and gastrointestinal side-effects, including headache, drowsiness, dizziness, cramps, bleeding of the stomach or intestines, diarrhoea and blood disorders. One pharmacopoeia, in fact, states that this drug is not superior to other mild analgesics (painkillers) and that there is no rational indication for its use. Yet doctors continue to prescribe it!

Thus, there is always a price to pay when we attempt to alter nature's processes by unnatural methods. Although the side-effects of medication and surgical intervention may not be immediately apparent, they usually make themselves known in the long term, sometimes in irreversible ways. Treatments compatible with nature may take longer to work and require a little more patience and persistence. But they do not undermine health. They enhance it.

## Signs and Symptoms

Problems associated with primary dysmenorrhoea may, for simplicity, be grouped loosely into three categories:

— those associated with fluid retention, such as swelling, breast tenderness and irritability:

— gastrointestinal (referring to the stomach and intestines) symptoms, such as nausea, vomiting and diarrhoea; and

— cramps and pain.

These symptoms may be experienced at any time from ovulation to the start of the menstrual flow. When they start with the menstrual flow, they are usually referred to as *dysmenorrhoea*, or difficult menstruation. When they occur between ovulation and the menstrual flow, the sufferer is said to be experiencing *Premenstrual Syndrome*, or PMS. (A syndrome is a collection of signs and symptoms characterizing a particular condition.)

Primary dysmenorrhoea may, again for convenience, be

classified as either spasmodic or congestive, depending on the signs and symptoms manifested.

## Spasmodic Dysmenorrhoea

Spasmodic dysmenorrhoea usually appears about two years after menstruation begins, that is, about the time ovulation starts. It most frequently occurs between the ages of fifteen and twenty-five, often ending dramatically after a full-term pregnancy, or gradually lessening in severity with each menstrual period, somewhere in the twenties.

In the days just before menstruation starts, the woman usually feels very well. With the onset of the period, however, she experiences spasmodic pain, which generally appears about every twenty minutes and lasts about five minutes—similar to labour pains. The pain occurs in the lower abdomen. It is sharp and colicky and may radiate to the thighs and lower back. It rarely lasts more than twenty-four hours.

It seems that this type of dysmenorrhoea is associated with an oestrogen level inadequate for maturing and stretching the uterine muscles. Perhaps that is why pregnancy, with its high oestrogen level and a growing foetus to stretch the walls of the uterus, often results in absence of pain once the periods recommence. High levels of prostaglandins also seem implicated in this type of dysmenorrhoea.

## Congestive Dysmenorrhoea

Congestive dysmenorrhoea and its related Premenstrual Syndrome, or PMS, can start as early as puberty and continue until menopause. Childbirth brings no relief. The condition seems to worsen following each pregnancy.

The greatest difficulty appears to be experienced in the week or so before menstruation starts. During this time, there can be dull, continuous pain in the lower abdomen. It increases in severity on the first day of menstruation, gradually diminishing as the period progresses. The pain seems to be aggravated by smoking and stress. Associated problems may be divided into two categories, as follows:

| *Psychological* | *Somatic* (physical) |
|---|---|
| Depression, crying spells and mood swings | Swelling of legs and fingers |
| Tension, anxiety and irritability | Bloated feeling in abdomen |
| Decreased energy and fatigue | Weight gain |
| Increased energy | Breast tenderness |
| Decreased or increased sexual desire | Heart palpitations |
| Feelings of irrationality or violence | Headaches and dizziness |
| Changes in eating habits | Excessive thirst and appetite |
| | Sleep disorders |
| | Constipation or diarrhoea |
| | Back pain |
| | Acne |
| | Clumsiness and minor accidents |

# CHAPTER 3

# Understanding Pain

A look at a medical dictionary will confirm that the word
*pain* comes from the Latin *poena*, which means a fine or
penalty. The Latin word in turn stems from the Sanskrit root
*pu*, meaning sacrifice.

In primitive societies when someone was in pain, she (or
he) was thought to be possessed by an evil spirit. To get rid
of the pain, the sufferer had to banish the spirit and this was
done through the use of charms or magic formulas. Later,
when pain was regarded as punishment (as suggested by the
Latin origin of the word) which had been meted out by some
offended god, attempts to eliminate it were made by offering
sacrifices and by the performance of elaborate rituals, as
propitiation to the wronged deity.

In present-day civilized societies, these views are seemingly
no longer held and yet, the degree of pain experienced is
influenced not only by physical factors, but also by religious
beliefs, ethnic background and personality. Memory, attention, fear and a host of other influences also play a part in
how we respond to pain stimuli.

**Toleration of Pain**
We sometimes wonder why certain people seem to tolerate
pain better than others. One plausible explanation lies in the
now-classic spinal 'gate control theory' of pain, proposed in
the 1960s by Ronald Melzack, a professor at McGill
University, Montreal, and Patrick Wall. They suggest that
there is a nervous mechanism that, in effect, opens or closes

a 'gate' controlling pain stimuli reaching the brain for interpretation. This mechanism can be affected by certain psychological processes; your attitude to an event can determine if you'll feel pain and how much. If you're anxious, it'll increase your perception of pain. If you're tense, you'll feel the pain more keenly. Your cultural heritage may also have a bearing. In one experiment, for example, northern Europeans reported feeling 'warm' while persons of Mediterranean origin complained of pain when subjected to the same source and degree of heat. More dramatically, people from certain societies in various parts of the world inflict wounds on themselves, without apparent pain, as they engage in 'rites of passage'. I can tell many tales concerning women of various nationalities in labour. My observations lead me to conclude that those from the Caribbean, Latin American countries, Italy and India, to name a few, tolerate pain less and are more vocal in their response to it than women from the British Isles, for example.

In his book, *Yoga and Medicine,* Dr Steven F. Brena (the Assistant Professor and Director of the Pain Division, Department of Anesthesiology and Anesthesia Research Center, University of Washington School of Medicine, Seattle) gives examples of how this spinal gate mechanism works:

Imagine that you're standing in a campground, holding a paper cup of hot coffee. You spill some and burn yourself. You drop the cup and shake your hand. Now pretend that you're in the home of your employer. In your hand you have an expensive china cup of tea. You again burn yourself. *You first put down the cup safely. Then you shake your hand.*

Why the different reactions? In the second example, when the burning sensation was relayed to the brain, you quickly *evaluated* the consequences of damaging your employer's expensive rug or breaking the china teacup. The emotional centres in your brain inhibited further painful sensations until *after* you put the cup down safely and avoided damaging the rug. In the first example, no such inhibition took place because, upon assessment, no harm could be seen to come either to the campground or to the paper cup you let fall.

This is in keeping with the spinal gate control theory. Simply, when the gate is 'open', painful impulses can get through to the brain where it is interpreted as pain. When the gate is 'closed', few or no sensations reach it. For instance, in cases where prisoners were able to withstand the suffering of prolonged torture by the enemy, the captives were able to close their spinal gates temporarily, as it were, to the entry of sensory inputs.

A similar occurrence manifests itself when a trained woman approaches childbirth. She has learned to relax between and with contractions. She has been taught to use her breath to full advantage. She perceives the sensations occurring in labour not as pain, but as pressure and stretching.

It may be interesting to make some observations here about placebos. A *placebo* is a non-pharmacological ('non-drug') agent given to please or satisfy a patient (the word originates from Latin and literally means, 'I shall please'). It may be considered a form of psychotherapy—a treating of the mind. I have seen patients who were becoming dependent on analgesics (painkillers) respond very well indeed to treatment with placebos. Some women suffering from dysmenorrhoea have also been treated with placebos. Mind over matter?

How can we close our spinal gate to shut out some of the painful stimuli reaching the brain and alter our mental evaluation of the hurt?

## Drugs
We can use analgesics or tranquillizers to dull emotional response. But these can produce undesirable reactions. Here, for your information, are a number of drugs currently used in treating PMS and dysmenorrhoea and some of their side-effects.

*Oestrogen-progestin combinations (oral contraceptives, or the Pill):* Nausea, vomiting, abdominal pain, diarrhoea, constipation, possible blood circulation disorders such as clots, high blood-pressure, headache, migraine, swelling, weight gain, vitamin $B_9$ (folic acid) deficiency—due to malabsorption generated by contraceptive pills, visual disorders, mood changes, altered menstrual pattern, tenderness and fullness of the breasts, increase in size of uterine tumours, skin discoloration.

*Diuretics ('water pills') to treat swelling by increasing urinary output of water and salt (sodium):* Weakness, leg cramps, dryness of the mouth, dizziness, disturbances of the stomach and intestines, confusion, low blood-pressure, lethargy, headache, malaise, abdominal pain, nausea, vomiting, breathing difficulties, heart irregularities, difficulty in speaking, etc. (In one pharmacopoeia, a whole page is devoted to the possible side-effects of diuretics!)

*Progestogens (synthetic compounds with progesterone-type activity):* Spotting of blood, irregular periods, nausea, lethargy, disturbances of the stomach and intestines, increase in body temperature, decreased sex drive, jaundice. High dosage may cause masculinization of the female foetus.

*Anti-depressants:* Restlessness, headache, dizziness, drowsiness, insomnia, constipation, loss of appetite (anorexia), urinary retention or frequency, swelling of hands and feet, anaemia. Long-term use occasionally causes damage to the eyes, flushing, increased perspiration, appetite stimulation and weight gain. High dosage may activate latent schizophrenia.

*Anti-anxiety agents:* Drowsiness, allergic reactions, blood disorders, dizziness, inability to urinate, headaches, nausea, vomiting, constipation, low blood-pressure, fainting spells, fever, breathing difficulties, weakness, emotional instability and confusion.

*Bromocriptine Mesylate (Parlodel), a non-hormonal agent used to treat PMS. It inhibits the release of the hormone prolactin by the pituitary gland:* High incidence (sixty-eight per cent) of mild adverse effects: nausea (fifty-one per cent), headaches (eight per cent), abdominal cramps (seven per cent), light-headedness (six per cent), vomiting (five per cent), nasal congestion (five per cent), constipation (three per cent) and slight lowering of blood-pressure.

*Danzol (Danocrine), a synthetic androgen (male sex hormone) that inhibits the release of FSH and LH by the pituitary gland. This arrests ovulation and menstruation (both usually resume 60-90 days after use of the drug is discontinued):* Weak symptoms of masculinization such as mild hirsutism (e.g. hair growth on face and chest), decreased breast size, deepening of the voice, oiliness of the skin. Also acne, swelling, weight gain, flushing, sweating, vaginal itching, nervousness and emotional instability.

The names of some prostaglandin synthetase inhibitors and their adverse effects have already been mentioned in Chapter 2 (page 22).

It is noteworthy, and not a little ironic, that many of these untoward symptoms are the very ones from which sufferers of PMS and dysmenorrhoea seek relief!

## Natural Pain Control

According to Dr Brena, everyone has the potential to limit, control or even prevent pain through will-power.

Natural pain control methods are largely based on 'closing the gate' so as to influence input from receptors reaching the brain. The beauty of these methods, compared with pharmacological approaches (i.e. medication), is that they produce no unsalutary side-effects. They mobilize the body's own natural resources to promote well-being.

The following are some currently used methods of natural pain relief.

## Acupuncture

The ancient Chinese practice of acupuncture involves inserting special needles into specific body sites and then twirling them manually. It is believed to work by stimulating certain large nerve fibres to prevent the 'gate from opening', by short-circuiting the usual transmission pathways. In several recent well controlled studies, acupuncture was shown to provide substantial relief of certain chronic pain states.

Professor Melzack has referred to acupuncture as a form of *hyperstimulation analgesia* (literally, pain relief through overstimulation) comparable with the old-fashioned practices of cupping or blistering the skin. To put it very simply: intense stimulation of trigger (or acupuncture) points seems to bring about pain relief by 'closing the gate' to inputs that would be interpreted by the brain as painful.

Recent Canadian research indicates that acupuncture also stimulates the release of *endorphins*. These are morphine-like substances occurring naturally in the brain; they act as the body's natural painkillers.

## Transcutaneous Electrical Nerve Stimulation

Also in this category is transcutaneous electrical nerve stimulation, recently found to be a powerful technique for the control of pain in the lower back, neck and head. When administered like acupuncture, for short periods of time, at moderate-to-high stimulation intensities (i.e. just below painful levels), it often produces relief from pain for hours, days or weeks.

You can carry out this procedure daily by yourself, at home, for gradually increasing pain relief, using an electronic device specially designed for this purpose. Called a transcutaneous nerve stimulator, it was introduced not long ago by a leading expert on pain, Dr C. Norman Shealy. It is described in Dr Harold Gelb's book entitled *Killing Pain Without Prescription*.

## Psychological Factors

Management of pain, long considered the almost exclusive province of those specializing in the structure and function of the human body (e.g. anatomists, physiologists and neurologists), now increasingly concerns psychologists. This is because, according to Professor Melzack, pain is profoundly affected by psychological factors such as anxiety, attention, prior conditioning, suggestion and personality variables.

New approaches to pain therapy therefore include hypnosis, various forms of psychotherapy, biofeedback and techniques involving distraction, visualization, breathing and relaxation.

## Biofeedback

There is convincing evidence that biofeedback is very effective in at least one kind of pain—tension headache. Through biofeedback, sufferers learn to relax the muscles of their forehead to reduce the tension contributing to the pain.

Used in combination with hypnosis, biofeedback has also produced significant relief of pain in a variety of other instances—a reminder that pain is multi-faceted, with sensory, affective (referring to mood and emotions) and evaluative components.

## Hypnosis

During the past two decades, there has been some success with hypnosis in the management of some chronic pain states. In these cases, the object is not only to control the pain itself but also to relieve the accompanying emotional distress. Hypnosis seems to meet these objectives, to some extent, in selected cases. It has the advantage of not producing unpleasant or destructive side-effects and it contributes as well to promoting life-enhancing attitudes.

Hypnosis, of course, has been successfully employed for some time in helping pregnant women cope with the discomfort and pain of labour. Since some forms of dysmenorrhoea are reminiscent of labour pains, it is not unreasonable to suppose that hypnosis may be useful in this area as well.

**Relaxation**

In his book, *You Must Relax*, researcher and psychiatrist Dr Edmund Jacobson describes the results of tests done on normal subjects. When exposed to a source of distress, such as a headache or pressure from a tight band applied around the forehead during the experiment, the subjects' nerve/muscle reactions registered overactivity. The same reaction occurs in cases of pain from inflamed or swollen tissues where sensory nerves are subjected to increased pressure or tension. Dr Jacobson has observed, however, that advanced relaxation tends to diminish certain types of pain.

According to Bruce Smollen, MD, and Brian Schulman, MD, authors of *Pain Control: The Bethesda Program*, genuine relaxation can actually lower the experience of pain. It works because it slows down the body's alerting, or sympathetic, response, thereby breaking the fear-tension-pain cycle. Mastery and daily practice of progressive deep muscle relaxation can greatly contribute to effective pain control. There are detailed instructions for just such a technique in Chapter 7. I have successfully taught this method to hundreds of students over the past decade. In a stress-management course that I have designed and instruct for the school district where I live, it is the highlight of each lesson. Students love the technique and have told me what a difference it makes to their general feeling of well-being. Please remember that the more relaxed you are, the less intensely you tend to feel pain.

**Breathing**

There is a close relationship between the perception of, and reaction to, pain and our respiratory (breathing) system. Dr Steven Brena explains that when someone experiences discomfort or pain, breathing usually speeds up and becomes irregular and difficult. When we talk about pain leaving us breathless, or pain 'knocking the wind' out of us, we acknowledge this connection.

If we therefore consciously slow down our breathing and make it more even (as far as circumstances permit), we can ease discomfort and pain considerably, lessen anxiety and tension and promote relaxation. This brings the pain under our own conscious, wilful control. We also provide ourselves with a mental diversion, so that we perceive the pain less intensely. This is one of the principles so successfully used in training women for childbirth. In Chapter 7, I have outlined in detail several excellent breathing techniques which I've taught for many years to innumerable students.

## Exercise

Studies have shown that people who exercise regularly tend to have an advantage over those who don't when it comes to coping with pain. In one study, Dr Lee S. Berk, a preventive health-care specialist at Loma Linda University Medical Centre in California, measured the endorphin levels in both athletes and sedentary persons. He found that those who exercised regularly produced greater amounts of endorphins during stressful situations, and that they also produced them more readily than those who neglected exercise.

An especially useful form of exercise for sufferers of difficult menstruation, and symptoms associated with it, is the slow-moving, stretching type done in synchronization with breathing. Dr Loren Fishman, of Albert Einstein College of Medicine in the USA, has reported an improvement in his patients to whom he prescribed such exercises, after about three months of faithful practice. I have selected and described in detail several such exercises in Chapter 6. I have taught these exercises to countless women for more than a decade, for the relief of a variety of conditions, including backache, headache and other difficulties in which tension was a significant contributing factor.

In addition to these exercises, brisk walking, swimming, bicycling, horseback riding or other safe form of aerobic type exercise (to stimulate the heart and lungs) is suggested, in the days preceding the onset of troublesome menstrual symptoms.

## Heat and Cold
The application of heat for pain relief is as old as the hills. Physiotherapists still frequently apply hot packs to their clients' painful joints and muscles, especially those of the neck and back, to give relief.

In one gynaecology ward where I worked, the Sister lent us a hot-water bottle and ordered us to bed when she sensed that we were suffering from menstrual cramps. The treatment invariably worked. When using a hot-water bottle, please remember to put a cover over it (an old pillow-case will do) to prevent burns to the skin. Some women also find comfort from an electric heating pad. It's best to keep this on the lowest possible setting to avoid the risk of burns.

The application of cold as a pain relief method is also very old. People still use ice-bags for some forms of headache and abdominal pain. Cold applied to swollen, painful areas (such as a joint or limb) will often bring relief. You can make a simple ice compress by soaking a piece of linen in iced water, wringing it out and laying it over the affected part.

In one maternity ward where I worked, the nurse in charge gave slim ice packs to women who had just given birth, to place at the episiotomy site to relieve swelling, discomfort and pain.

## Massage
Manual massage is useful for some forms of pain because it promotes good blood circulation to the affected part and reduces tension. Gentle, light stroking—a sort of *effleurage*, such as that used to ease back and abdominal discomfort during labour—is sometimes an effective relief measure for other types of pain.

Another interesting form of massage is done with what is known as an intra-sound (as opposed to ultra-sound) massager, now available in some health food stores. The appliance, which is lightweight and looks like a shower head, consists of a hand-held transducer that produces vibration of a 'soundhead' for external application to the body.

The intra-sound massager is useful for the temporary relief of muscle and joint pain and some types of headache, to mention just two. It is *not* recommended for use by epileptics, those experiencing pain due to internal infection or persons with pacemakers.

One wonders why, with such a wealth of natural pain relievers from which to choose, there is still so much dependency on medication. Perhaps it is because it is so fast and easy to swallow a pill. Natural methods do take a little longer to work; but they don't produce deleterious side-effects which must surely be a strong point in their favour.

# CHAPTER 4

# Diet for a Symptom-free Menstrual Cycle: Part I

Many experts now believe that the monthly hormonal changes that occur in a woman's body contribute to certain nutritional deficiencies or imbalances. They believe that these aberrations underlie the distressing signs and symptoms associated with PMS and dysmenorrhoea. Chief among the nutrients implicated are sodium (salt), pyridoxine (vitamin $B_6$), glucose (sugar) and magnesium.

However, all nutrients have a synergic or 'working together' action. Therefore, a number of other nutrients, e.g. calcium, iron and the entire vitamin B-complex are involved, and these—and others—will be considered.

## Sodium (salt)

One of the most outstanding signs of PMS is oedema, or swelling. This is usually due to water retention, which is in turn associated with too much salt in the tissues. A hormonal imbalance, in which progesterone levels are low relative to oestrogen levels, is thought to contribute to the premenstrual swelling experienced by many women. Progesterone is a natural diuretic which facilitates the excretion of surplus fluid and sodium from body tissues.

When progesterone levels are inadequate, there is increased sodium and water retention in the body. This produces such symptoms as tension, fatigue, weight gain, joint pain, a feeling of bloatedness and swelling. The swelling is not always confined to the hands and feet. Some women experience swelling of the face and eyelids. Others report an inability to wear their contact lenses because of increased intraocular (within the eye) pressure due to accumulated fluid. Still others report visual disturbances.

Apart from its relationship to swelling, sodium retention has been associated with another PMS symptom—depression. Clinical studies have shown a significant decrease in body sodium content following recovery from depression. Also, depressed subjects treated with lithium (an element involved in sodium metabolism and its transportation in nerves and muscles) showed changes in sodium distribution in the body, because of marked elimination of sodium through urination.

As remedy, doctors frequently prescribe diuretics ('water pills') which work by helping rid the body of surplus fluid. But diuretics also cause the excretion of important substances, particularly potassium, a mineral element vital to many body functions such as the maintenance of acid-base balance, normal excitability of heart muscle and conduction of nerve impulses. (Acid-base balance is a term used to refer to the mechanisms by which the acids and alkalies are kept in a state of equilibrium.)

Yet despite evidence that the adverse effects of diuretics far outweigh their benefits (see page 29), doctors continue to prescribe these 'water pills'. Moreover, the non-specific action of many of these diuretics may actually aggravate PMS by promoting a deficiency of important minerals, e.g. potassium and magnesium.

## Function of sodium

Sodium is necessary to preserve a balance between calcium and potassium to maintain normal heart action and the equilibrium of the body. Sodium, potassium and chlorine are important in keeping body fluids near neutrality. They determine the amount of fluid held in body tissues; they attract nutrients from the intestines into the blood, and from the blood into the cells, by maintaining what is known as osmotic pressure; and they are essential components of glandular secretions.

## Reducing salt intake naturally

It is a mistake to think that if sodium is so important to the healthful functioning of the body, ingesting large amounts would be beneficial. Many women, in fact, consume twenty to fifty times the amount of salt they need daily.

One of the first steps to take toward reducing your salt intake is to become a seasoned label-reader. As you shop, scrutinize labels for the presence of salt in the products you plan to purchase. Look for the words 'salt', 'soda' and 'sodium'.

Salt is found in many guises. Some of the most common sodium-containing additives found in commercially prepared foods are: sodium ascorbate, sodium benzoate, sodium caseinate, sodium citrate, sodium EDTA, sodium nitrate, sodium metabisulfate and monosodium glutamate (MSG). Products marked 'no salt added' or 'made without salt' are not necessarily low in sodium. Carefully read the ingredient listing before deciding to purchase. Additives collectively referred to as stabilizers, emulsifiers and preservatives are also likely to contain sodium.

A safe general rule, then, is to avoid, as far as is practicable, habitually using highly processed, packaged foods. Be selective, too, of the brand of mineral water you routinely use. Some brands are high in sodium.

## Sensible seasonings

Most foods contain their own natural salt. In many cases, you don't need to add salt to food either when cooking it or when about to eat it.

Experiment with culinary herbs (available at herbalists, health food stores and most supermarkets). Dried herbs have about twice the strength of fresh: 2ml (½ teaspoon) dried herb is equivalent to 5ml (1 teaspoon) fresh. It is usual to add the former to the pot during the last hour or so of the cooking period.

*Note well:* avoid using herb salts, e.g. garlic salt and celery salt. They're high in sodium. Instead, use the fresh or dehydrated counterpart, e.g a clove of fresh garlic or garlic flakes. A small ceramic mortar and pestle is useful for grinding seeds for a fresher flavour (e.g. celery seeds) than that imparted by already-ground seasonings. For nutmeg, use the finest perforations on a standard grater, and for pepper use a peppermill. The flavour of freshly ground peppercorns is superior to bottled ground black or white pepper. For most herbs, the general rule is: a little goes a long way.

Some herbs to use as salt alternatives are: basil, bouquet garni, celery seed, chervil, chives, coriander, cumin, dill, fennel, fines herbes, marjoram, mint, oregano, paprika, parsley, rosemary, saffron, savoury, tarragon and thyme. (A natural 'herb salt' recipe is included in chapter 11 page 178.)

### Other low-salt hints

Drastically reduce, or eliminate altogether, your consumption of cured meats such as bacon, ham, pepperoni and salami. Severely restrict your intake of salty snacks such as salted crackers and nuts, potato chips, pretzels and pickles. Instead, eat fresh fruit and raw, fresh vegetables (celery, though, is high in sodium), freshly shelled nuts, whole grain (unsalted) crackers and crispbreads and home-made yogurt (you'll find a recipe on page 180).

Substitute freshwater fish like carp, mullet, pike and whitefish for the salty varieties. Eat spinach sparingly; it has a high sodium content.

### Natural diuretics

In addition to curbing your salt intake, you may use the following natural diuretics without fear of untoward reactions: cranberry juice, kelp, parsley, watercress.

Refer also to Chapter 8 for herbs with diuretic properties.

### Pyridoxine (Vitamin B$_6$)

Researchers have found that some women experiencing PMS have elevated prolactin levels. *Prolactin* is a hormone produced by the anterior lobe of the pituitary gland (located in the brain). It is involved, with other hormones such as oestrogen and progesterone, in the lactation process (referring to milk secretion). But it has other metabolic functions as well, some of which are not yet fully understood.

High doses of pyridoxine have, according to reports, depressed prolactin levels sufficiently to effect relief from the symptoms they apparently produce. Studies have shown that, in women suffering from PMS because of high oestrogen in relation to progesterone levels, the hormonal imbalance produced a pyridoxine deficiency that responded well to supplementation with this nutrient.

## The role of pyridoxine

Pyridoxine is required to regulate hormonal activity. It aids proper food assimilation. It is necessary for the production of antibodies which protect from infection and aids in the formation of red blood cells. It is important for the proper functioning of the nervous system, including the brain cells. Pyridoxine plays an essential role in the synthesis of important neurotransmitters (chemical substances facilitating transmission of nerve impulses). It activates many enzyme systems. It protects against degenerative disease processes such as diabetes and some forms of heart disease. *It has also been used as a natural diuretic* to relieve premenstrual oedema.

Pyridoxine plays an important part in protein metabolism. Our requirement for this nutrient varies directly with our protein intake, and popular high protein diets therefore increase our need for it.

Pyridoxine also has an important role in fat (lipid) metabolism, particularly that of the essential fatty acids. In carbohydrate metabolism, pyridoxine helps to convert glycogen in the liver and muscles into glucose (sugar) for a ready source of energy to all cells. According to Sandra Cohen-Rose and Dr Colin Penfield Rose, co-authors of *The New Canadian High Energy Diet*, the low blood sugar levels that occur with pyridoxine deficiency are evidence of the role played by this nutrient in carbohydrate metabolism.

Pyridoxine helps to regulate the balance between the minerals sodium and potassium in the body—of great importance to vital body functions. It is needed for the proper absorption of vitamin $B_{12}$ and for the production of hydrochloric acid, a normal constituent of gastric (stomach) juice.

## Pyridoxine deficiency symptoms

These include anaemia ('iron-poor blood'), low blood sugar, oedema, mental depression, nervousness, irritability, insomnia (inability to sleep), migraine headaches and skin disorders—in short, symptoms characteristic of PMS.

## Encouraging results

A pioneer in clinical studies of pyridoxine, Dr John M. Ellis of Mt Pleasant, Texas, reports consistent success with this vitamin in treating women with severe premenstrual oedema.

In his book entitled *Vitamin $B_6$: The Doctor's Report,* Dr Ellis records the encouraging results obtained in treating women with between 50 and 100mg of pyridoxine daily for the relief of various forms of oedema. In several of these women, diuretics had failed to bring the desired results.

In several recent medical investigations, positive responses have been obtained in relieving fifty to sixty per cent of the symptoms characterizing PMS by daily administration of 100mg pyridoxine for one to two weeks prior to the menstrual flow. British researcher Dr G. D. Kerr has reported that pyridoxine is effective and well tolerated. It alleviates several PMS symptoms, especially irritability and depression.

Unlike diuretics, the possible adverse effects of which are myriad, and unlike hormones and the prolactin inhibitor bromocriptine (see Chapter 3), pyridoxine produces virtually no untoward symptoms and poses no long-term risk, even with dosages as high as 200mg daily.

Many other therapists have successfully used pyridoxine to treat PMS. Two of them, Dr Guy E. Abraham (formerly of the UCLA School of Medicine, Harbor General Hospital, Torrance, California) and Dr Joel T. Hargrove (of Rolling Hills, California) have reported significant behavioural improvement in more than eighty per cent of women treated with this vitamin. Another doctor, P. W. Adams of St Mary's Hospital School in London, England, found that after treating emotionally distressed women with 20mg pyridoxine twice daily, they improved significantly. These women had been using oral contraceptive pills which increase pyridoxine needs by as much as 30mg per day. By increasing pyridoxine intake, symptoms like the depression associated with the use of oral contraceptives can be relieved. This type of depression has been attributed to the body's failure to convert tryptophan (a protein) to serotonin, a neurotransmitter in the brain. Even women who do not habitually use oral contraceptives have responded favourably to treatment with pyridoxine (refer to Dr Ellis's book, previously cited).

In addition, a Dr Leonard Snider has reported encouraging results in treating teenagers suffering from acne flare-ups prior to menstruation. They responded well to daily supplementation of 50mg pyridoxine.

## Dosage of vitamin $B_6$

The minimum daily requirement of pyridoxine for healthy adults is 2mg.

However, therapeuticaly, up to 200mg have been prescribed for several months, usually in combination with other B-complex vitamins. Treatment is best supervised by a competent therapist.

## Natural pyridoxine sources

Good natural sources of this important vitamin include the following: avocados, broccoli (raw), bananas, blackstrap molasses, buckwheat flour, cabbage, cantaloupe melons, cauliflower (raw), carrots, egg yolks, hazelnuts (filberts), green beans, green leafy vegetables, green peppers, milk, mushrooms (raw), oranges, peanuts, soyabean flour, marrow (squash), strawberries, sunflower seeds, walnuts, wheat bran, wheatgerm and nutritional yeast. Particularly rich sources of pyridoxine are—nutritional yeast, pecan nuts, potatoes, salmon, raw vegetables and whole grains.

The milling of grains leads to pyridoxine losses, sometimes as high as ninety per cent. Unfortunately, the law does not require that processed cereals be enriched with this nutrient. Also, freezing vegetables can reduce their pyridoxine content by as much as twenty-five per cent.

Pyridoxine is not destroyed by heat or acid, but by oxidation, alkali and ultraviolet light. It is therefore important to store and cook foods properly to keep such losses to a minimum. Good rules to follow, then, are: *don't* cut fruits and vegetables and leave them exposed to air, *don't* overcook vegetables or cook them in large amounts of water and then discard the cooking liquid, and *never* add bicarbonate of soda (baking soda) to vegetables to preserve their natural colour.

## Glucose (sugar)

Many of the troublesome signs and symptoms typical of PMS are due to an upset in the delicate balance between the levels of two hormones: oestrogen and progesterone. Even if progesterone levels are adequate for a symptom-free menstrual cycle, an excess of oestrogen will alter the oestrogen-progesterone balance and generate problems.

The effect of progesterone on glucose (sugar) metabolism can be pronounced. Without adequate progesterone, the body cannot metabolize sugar properly and a condition known as *hypoglycaemia* occurs. This means, simply, that there's a deficiency of sugar in the blood. It is sometimes referred to as 'low blood sugar'.

## Symptoms of hypoglycaemia

Hypoglycaemia is responsible for many of the perplexing and enervating symptoms of PMS, which are also characteristic of low blood sugar. These include acute fatigue, restlessness, general malaise, a loathing of one's daily routine, headache, irritability, hunger, weakness and a craving for sweets. In more severe cases, mental disturbances occur.

Numerous laboratory tests and physical examinations of over 900 persons who were too emotionally ill to work revealed no other abnormality than slightly low blood sugar levels. These individuals were depressed, had no interest in, or energy for, their daily tasks and had lost their joy of living. But, when given a diet adequate in protein, and snacks of milk and toast, improvement was dramatic and long-lasting. Moreover, therapy for those undergoing psychoanalysis was shortened.

This diet, which included no soft drinks or alcoholic beverages, is in effect the anti-hypoglycaemia diet described later in this chapter, page 47.

## The stress of low blood sugar

Some years ago, a baffling plane crash occurred. Investigators were puzzled because the pilot was very experienced, weather conditions were ideal and the aircraft itself was mechanically sound. Finally, the cause was found: the pilot was suffering from hypoglycaemia. This cast light on several other hitherto unexplained flying accidents. It became evident that the times of these mishaps coincided with those times when the pilots' blood sugar levels were lowest.

The blood sugar level after a night's fast (before breakfast) is quite low. Physicians regard it as 'basal', which is low enough to cause lack of energy—despite a good night's rest—feelings of listlessness, impatience, irritability, nausea, dizziness, faintness, slow reflexes, headache and even confusion in many people.

If you're one of these persons, and you start your day with

tea or coffee, with or without a doughnut or toast and jam or marmalade, or any breakfast made up largely of refined carbohydrates, you run the risk of setting in motion a potentially hazardous sequence of events. The blood sugar level rises temporarily; the body responds by sending insulin (a hormone secreted by the pancreas) into the bloodstream to metabolize the sugar; one and one-half or two hours later the blood sugar level plunges lower than basal level. You may experience some of the symptoms just mentioned, or you may faint. You may be driving and need to brake suddenly to avoid hitting a pedestrian or a dog. Adrenalin (a hormone secreted by the adrenal glands located above the kidneys) pours into your system in response to the stress of the situation. Increased metabolic demands force the blood sugar level farther downward. Think of the dire consequences if you're in any situation where keen concentration, crystal-clear thinking and sharp reflexes are vital. Think of how easily a reasonable discussion could turn into a heated argument and even into violence. It has happened.

If, on the other hand, you were to have with your tea or coffee and toast a piece of cheese, an egg, or porridge with milk, you could largely prevent a dramatic change in blood sugar level. Protein and complex carbohydrates ('slowly digested') stay in the system longer, and metabolize more slowly, than the highly processed carbohydrates that many persons routinely consume for breakfast.

Many people claim that they never feel hungry 'first thing in the morning' because of a huge meal eaten the night before. A study of the eating habits of overweight individuals who could not lose weight showed that they ate little throughout the day, made up for the deficit at dinnertime and had no appetite for breakfast. In the morning, the blood sugar level in these individuals is still fairly high from the meal eaten the evening before. They merely sample breakfast and lunch. Suddenly, the blood sugar level plunges and the symptoms of hypoglycaemia (mentioned earlier) begin to appear. The problem is not that too much, but rather too little, was eaten during the course of the day.

Skipping lunch can be almost as bad as missing breakfast. Dr J. Edgar Monagle, who has worked for many years as an expert in clinical nutrition with Canada's Department of National Health and Welfare, states that missing lunch is almost as common as going without breakfast—and only slightly less dangerous. He points out that after an interval of five or six hours between meals, physiological changes similar to those occurring after an overnight fast take place. He suggests that everyone who is engaged in work requiring keen concentration, alertness and reliable mental and physical responses, should not let more than four or so hours elapse between meals.

## The anti-hypoglycaemia diet

Many therapists and clinics are now recommending to clients suffering from PMS what they refer to as a 'standard hypoglycaemia diet'. I call it the anti-hypoglycaemia diet and this is what, basically, it embraces:

— Six smaller meals, compared with the usual three large, in a twenty-four-hour period. Three of the meals are moderate in size and three are essentially snacks taken in between.

— Neither fasting nor skipping of meals is permitted.

— Overprocessed and highly refined foods, e.g. white flour and white sugar, are contraindicated.

— Alcoholic beverages and products containing caffeine, e.g. coffee and cola drinks, are prohibited.

— Women troubled by swelling are advised to restrict their salt intake (see section on *sodium*, page 37).

In a nutshell, the anti-hypoglycaemia diet consits predominantly of protein foods and complex ('slowly digested') carbohydrates. These take a little longer to be converted into glucose, thereby providing the bloodstream with a continuous supply of glucose. They are also richer in minerals and vitamins and other essential nutrients than highly processed foods.

The following is a basic list of foods to eat and those to avoid. For recipes, please refer to Chapter 11.

| *Foods to eat* | *Foods to avoid* |
| --- | --- |
| Whole grains and whole grain products | White flour, white sugar and polished white rice |
| Nuts (fresh from the shell) and seeds | 'Pop', cordials and synthetic fruit-flavoured drinks |
| Milk and milk products | Cakes, pastries and doughnuts |
| Eggs | Salted nuts, crackers, potato crisps and pretzels |
| Fish | |
| Legumes (dried peas, beans and lentils) | Jams |
| Fresh fruits in season | Most brands of commercially prepared cold breakfast cereals |
| Fresh vegetables (restrict celery, if on a low-salt regimen) | Sherbert, jelly, ice cream, tinned fruits in syrup or otherwise sweetened |
| Green leafy vegetables (restrict spinach if on a low-salt regimen) | Tinned puddings |
| Naturally sweetened fruit juices | Sweets and chocolate |
| Freshly pressed vegetable juices | Many brands of cake mix |

## Hidden sugars

It is estimated that the amount of sugar many people consume through the habitual use of packaged foods is about 13.5kg or approximately 30 pounds. These 'hidden sugars', derived from corn syrup, refined sugar and other such sweeteners, are found abundantly in many common processed foods. For example, twenty per cent of a leading brand of tomato ketchup is sugar; thirty per cent of a popular brand of Russian salad dressing is sugar; sixty-five per cent of a well-known coffee whitener is sugar!

When shopping, read labels carefully. Remember that ingredients are listed in the order in which they predominate.

For example, in a product carrying this listing: Water, beef, sodium, spices; water accounts for most of the weight. Look out for sugar under various names, e.g. sucrose, dextrose and lactose. Many brands of commercially prepared cold breakfast cereals are essentially sugar. Some contain as much as seventy per cent!

## Sweet pitfalls

We do not have to rely on refined sugar to give us energy. Almost every food in its original form contains natural sugar or starch (which is changed into simple sugar by the body). Even if you don't touch a granule of sugar, you can obtain as much as two cups of it per day from the foods you eat.

The more refined the sugar you eat, the more rapid the destruction of the B vitamins (vital for superb health), and the greater your body's need for these nutrients. Refined sugar gives only a temporary increase of energy; in an hour or two, your blood sugar level will plunge to a level too low for well-being.

Be aware that much brown sugar is actually white sugar with molasses added. Use even unrefined raw cane sugar sparingly. Sweeten your baked goods with unrefined honey, molasses, dates or other dried fruits. Whatever the supposed merits of the sweetener of choice, however, use it discriminately.

Alternatives to sweets can include: seeds (e.g. sunflower, sesame, pumpkin); nuts (peanuts, almonds, walnuts, hazelnuts, Brazil nuts, pistachios, pecans—unsalted—and 'soy nuts', made from soybeans); and sun-dried fruits, eaten after a main meal. Brush your teeth immediately afterwards.

## Sweet nothings

About two hundred years ago, the average individual in affluent countries such as ours consumed less than a kilogram (about two pounds) of sugar a year. This commodity was sold mainly in pharmacies and treated as a drug. Today, the average person in many countries in the Western world consumes about 50kg (approximately 110 pounds) of sugar a year, that is, about 1kg (2.2 pounds) a week. This includes sugar ingested not only in beverages, but also in many other food items that seem to be an inseparable part of today's living, e.g. barbecue sauces, ketchup, and tinned beans, fruit and soups.

Refined sugar is a 'non-food'. It provides empty calories. It can produce nutrient deficiencies because, as it is metabolized, it uses up essential nutrients particularly the B vitamins. Excessive sugar intake has been implicated in the rise of obesity, coronary heart disease, adult-onset diabetes, hypoglycaemia and dental caries.

There is therefore no advantage in consuming as much sugar as many of us do. This applies as well to raw sugar. Pancake syrups and other syrups on the market are essentially sugar and water. Rather than habitually use them, try yogurt and fruit as alternative toppings. Honey, organic or otherwise, does contain traces of some minerals and vitamins, but not enough to warrant excessive consumption. It is, after all, a sweetener and all sweeteners can contribute to malnutrition unless used moderately, because they replace more healthful foods.

Watch out for imitation maple syrups, which are merely cane or corn syrup with added simulated maple flavouring and preservatives. These usually say 'maple flavoured syrup' on the labels.

Don't programme your taste buds to expect large quantities of sweetener, low-calorie or otherwise. Gradually cut down where you can. Omit frostings and icings from cakes. Reduce the sugar called for in most recipes for baked goods, beverages, puddings and sauces. In short, start a sweetness de-programming campaign.

## Magnesium

Researchers have found significantly lower levels of magnesium in women with PMS than in those not suffering from the syndrome. They attribute this to either a stress-induced decrease in magnesium absorption, or to increased urinary excretion of the mineral. The resulting magnesium deficiency would account for many of the physical and behavioural symptoms typical of PMS.

Guy E. Abraham, M.D., a former professor of obstetrics and gynaecology at the UCLA School of Medicine in California, and a colleague, Michael M. Lubran, M.D., Ph.D., made a study of twenty-six women suffering from premenstrual tension. They found that these women had significantly lower red blood cell levels of magnesium than did their asymptomatic (without symptoms) counterparts who served as controls. (Magnesium stays largely inside blood cells while the quantity in the plasma—the liquid part of blood—varies little.)

Dr Abraham and his colleague further noted that many of the symptoms of premenstrual tension were very similar to classic stress symptoms. They suggest that premenstrual tension may induce depletion of the body's magnesium stores, and that the symptoms of premenstrual tension may be due to magnesium deficiency—a vicious circle.

## Success with magnesium supplementation

Some doctors who prescribe magnesium supplements report a high success rate in treating PMS sufferers, regardless of the nature of the symptoms—mental or physical. Stress seems to cause increased magnesium excretion from the body, as well as decreased magnesium absorption. In addition, if the diet is high in sugar, fat and alcohol and low in fresh vegetables, it aggravates this state of magnesium deficiency.

A recent survey (based on the Canadian National Center for Health Statistics data) revealed that about fourteen per cent of teenage girls often miss school because of dysmenorrhoea, cramps being the leading cause of absenteeism. Magnesium has brought relief, even in cases where powerful painkillers like codeine have failed.

**Daily Dosage of Magnesium**

According to the late Paavo Airola, N.D., Ph.D., the daily recommended dosage of magnesium for non-pregnant women is 350mg, and the best form of supplement is magnesium chloride. However, therapeutic doses may go as high as 700mg daily. It is best, of course, to have supervision by a competent therapist.

According to the late Adelle Davis, one of America's best known nutritionists, the average daily magnesium requirement for healthy non-pregnant women is about 500mg. She points out, however, that this dosage gives a bare margin over the amounts lost daily in urine, faeces (stool) and perspiration.

Magnesium requirement is proportionate to calcium intake. The more the latter in the diet, the more the need of the former; and calcium given alone can induce magnesium deficiency. The correct proportion of these two nutrients seems to be approximately twice as much calcium as magnesium, that is, 500mg magnesium for every 1000mg calcium. Health food stores sell tablets containing the proper proportions, e.g. dolomite. Various other forms of magnesium supplement, e.g. magnesium carbonate and magnesium chloride, have been successfully used in combating deficiencies.

Some doctors suggest taking magnesium along with pyridoxine. Pyridoxine enhances the effect of magnesium. It is not well absorbed unless magnesium is well supplied in the diet. The lack of either nutrient may produce the same symptoms.

*Functions of magnesium*

Magnesium, according to Sandra Cohen-Rose and Dr Colin Penfield Rose, is important in many biological reactions, especially those involving nerve and muscle functions. Adelle Davis has referred to magnesium as 'nature's own tranquillizer'. It is needed by every cell in the body, the brain cells included. Magnesium is essential for the synthesis of proteins, the utilization of carbohydrates and fats and is an important catalyst (helper) in many enzyme reactions, particularly energy production.

Magnesium helps in the utilization of the B-complex vitamins (including pyridoxine), vitamin E, fats, calcium and other minerals. As well as this it is needed for healthy muscle tone and sound bones; it is essential for a healthy heart; it regulates the acid-alkaline balance in the body; and it plays a part in regulating female hormones. *It is a natural diuretic*. Magnesium helps prevent a build-up of cholesterol and so protects against atherosclerosis. It is associated with the regulation of body temperature.

## Symptoms of magnesium deficiency

In her book entitled *Let's Eat Right to Keep Fit*, Adelle Davis presents convincing documentation to support the observation that persons only slightly deficient in magnesium become irritable, highly-strung, sensitive to noise, hyperexcitable, apprehensive and belligerent. Fortunately, she points out, improvement of symptoms is usually dramatic within hours after magnesium is taken.

Magnesium deficiency is apparently difficult to detect because, as mentioned earlier, the nutrient stays largely inside the blood cells while the quantity in the plasma varies little. Magnesium has been found to be unusually low in the blood cells of persons using diuretics and antibiotics.

Magnesium deficiency can result in loss of potassium and calcium from the body. It can lead to kidney stones and kidney damage, muscle cramps, heart attack, epileptic seizures, impaired protein metabolism, premature wrinkles and the nervous system symptoms already mentioned.

Magnesium deficiency symptoms have been produced in volunteers consuming fare typically ingested daily by millions of persons in so-called civilized countries: polished white rice, pasta made from refined flours, sweets, jams, baked goods made with white flour and soft drinks such as 'pop' and synthetic fruit drinks.

Adelle Davis has remarked that the principal reason why doctors write millions of prescriptions for tranquillizers each year is the nervousness, grouchiness and 'jitters' largely brought on by inadequate diets lacking magnesium. One of her colleagues, a psychiatrist, reported that after insisting that those with whom she was working improve their diets, so as to ensure adequate magnesium and calcium intake, she found not only that tranquillizers were no longer needed, but also that psychotherapy progressed more rapidly. Nature, they concluded, does provide her own tranquillizers.

## Natural magnesium sources

The best natural sources of this very important mineral include alfalfa sprouts, almonds (and other nuts eaten fresh from the shell), beetroot tops, brown rice, celery, chard, dried fruits, grapefruit, green leafy vegetables (particularly kale) grown on mineral rich soils, oranges, potatoes, sesame seeds, shellfish, soyabeans, sunflower seeds, wheat bran, wheatgerm and whole grains.

The milling of grains has reduced our magnesium intake considerably. White flour, for example, has only about twenty-two per cent of the magnesium found in wholewheat flour. The bran and germ of wheat—valuable sources of this nutrient—are removed during milling.

# CHAPTER 5

# Diet for a Symptom-free Menstrual Cycle: Part II

Fred Rohé, author of *The Complete Book of Natural Foods*, likens vitamins to the match that ignites an imaginary fire burning in our body. In this fire, the logs would be complex carbohydrates (starches and sugars), while protein and fat and the enzymes would be kindling. Yet without the match—the vitamins—nothing would happen. Vitamins are substances needed, in small amounts usually, to promote health and growth.

**The Water Soluble Vitamins**
These include vitamin C and the B vitamins (thiamin, riboflavin, niacin, pyridoxine, pantothenic acid, folacin, cobalamin and biotin).

Possibly the most prevalent nutrient deficiency is that of folacin. The milling of whole grains largely accounts for this (up to seventy-five per cent), as well as for other B vitamin losses. Only the 'Big Three' (thiamin, riboflavin and niacin) are added to white flour.

**The B Vitamins**
These are a complex of over twenty vitamins, often termed the 'nerve vitamins'. They cannot be stored in the body for any length of time. They are therefore a daily essential for the normal functioning of every cell and for maintaining a healthy nervous system. The entire group—the B-complex vitamins—is to be found in brewer's yeast and wheatgerm.

The B vitamins are highly synergistic. When using an

isolated B vitamin for therapeutic purposes, therefore, it is advisable to supplement with the entire complex to prevent imbalances occurring.

The greatest B-complex antagonists (literally, acting against) are coffee, contraceptive pills, alcohol, sleeping pills, tobacco, excessive sugar intake, stress and the over-cooking of foods.

Apart from pyridoxine (vitamin $B_6$) which was dealt with in Chapter 4, the following are notes on some of the vitamins that make up this complex.

## Thiamin (vitamin $B_1$)

Thiamin enables body cells to obtain energy from nutrients brought them through the blood circulation. It is sometimes called the 'morale vitamin'.

A thiamin deficiency can lead to loss of appetite, muscular weakness, shortness of breath, fatigue, irritability and oedema.

The richest sources of this vitamin are Brazil nuts, green leafy vegetables, legumes (dried beans, peas, lentils and peanuts), mushrooms, brewer's yeast (not to be confused with baker's yeast), potatoes, rolled oats, whole grains and yellow cornmeal.

An interesting fact about thiamin is that onions and garlic help it to be more readily absorbed. A substance called alliin, found in onion and garlic oils, combines with thiamin to form a compound known as allithiamine, which is very readily utilized.

Thiamin is easily destroyed by high heat and by alkalis. So when you toast your bread, for example, you reduce its thiamin content by one third.

## Riboflavin (vitamin $B_2$)

Riboflavin is essential for general good health. When riboflavin-deficient diets were fed to experimental subjects, symptoms including hypochondriasis (abnormal anxiety about one's health), depression, hysteria and weakness were produced.

Sunlight and ultraviolet light reduce the riboflavin content of food. It is wise, then, to purchase milk in opaque containers. Milk exposed to sunlight for two hours, for example, loses half its riboflavin content.

Good sources of this nutrient include cheese, lentils, milk (including evaporated), mushrooms, brewer's yeast and whole grains. (Four large or ten small mushrooms, by the way, yield 460 micrograms of riboflavin.)

A riboflavin deficiency can result in anaemia, various inflammations and eczema.

Both thiamin and riboflavin are found in these foods: asparagus, buckwheat flour, cantaloupe melons, green leafy vegetables, cod, lobsters, brewer's yeast, oranges, oysters, prunes, salmon, soya flour, turbot, wheatgerm and whole grains.

## Niacin (vitamin $B_3$)

Niacin is required for healthy blood circulation and a strong nervous system.

A niacin deficiency can produce irritability, nervousness, forgetfulness, headaches, digestive disorders, insomnia and depression. It can cause a condition called 'the four Ds', characterized by a progression from diarrhoea, depression, dementia (deteriorated mental state) to death.

In studies done on volunteers, niacin-deficient diets produced suspicious behaviour, cowardice, apprehension and mental confusion in subjects who were ordinarily strong, positive persons. A niacin deficiency was also shown to produce such undesirable traits as emotional instability, inability to co-operate and varying degrees of depression, ranging from mild 'blues' to a definite inability to cope with life's tougher situations.

Good niacin sources are: artichokes, asparagus, bass, cod, eggs, legumes, mushrooms, milk, brewer's yeast, nuts, peanut butter, peas, potatoes, rice bran, salmon, sunflower seeds, trout, tuna, wheat bran, whole grains and whole grain flours and yellow corn and its by-products.

*Caution:* excessive niacin intake can result in severe flushing and itching. Exercise caution when taking any B vitamin supplements.

## Folacin (vitamin B₉)

Folacin is imperative for healthy red blood cells and for keeping the body's natural defence mechanism in good working order. As already mentioned, some nutritionists believe that it is the nutrient most deficient in our diets.

A folacin deficiency can produce anaemia, skin disorders, impaired blood circulation and depression. Women on oestrogen contraceptive pills, and those whose alcohol intake is high, can easily suffer from a folacin deficiency unless an extra amount of the nutrient is taken.

Folacin comes from the Latin word for leaf, and so it is not surprising that its richest sources include intensely green leafy vegetables such as beetroot and turnip tops, lettuce and spinach. Fruits, potatoes and nuts are other good sources.

Folacin losses through cooking vegetables in too much water (and then discarding the liquid) and at high temperatures range from fifty to ninety per cent!

## Cobalamin (vitamin B₁₂)

This vitamin is essential for the production and regeneration of red blood cells and as a preventive against anaemia. A deficiency will lead to anaemia, symptoms of which include shortness of breath, fatigue and weakness. It can also result in nerve tissue degeneration.

Good food sources of cobalamin include eggs, milk and tempeh. Tempeh, pronounced 'tempay', is a staple food of Indonesia. It is made from hulled, split soyabeans that have been put through a process similar to yogurt making. The finished product has a consistency similar to that of a firm cake, with a flavour reminiscent of a cross between chicken and mushrooms. It is a high-protein, low-fat food which, like tofu, may be used as a meat alternative.

Because cobalamin is an 'animal' vitamin, vegans (vegetarians who use no animal products, eggs, milk or milk products) should take a vitamin B$_{12}$ supplement. But *please check* with a competent nutrition specialist.

This vitamin is destroyed by heat and light.

## Choline

Choline combines with another B vitamin to form lecithin, a fat-like substance produced daily by the liver, provided that these vitamins are amply supplied and the diet is otherwise adequate. Choline also helps to keep the arteries (blood vessels) elastic.

A choline deficiency contributes to high blood-pressure, liver disorders, hardening of the arteries, headaches, insomnia and constipation.

The richest sources of this nutrient are egg yolk, green leafy vegetables, brewer's yeast and wheatgerm.

## Pantothenic acid (calcium pantothenate)

This nutrient is essential for all body processes requiring energy, and for the health of every body cell. It has often been called the 'anti-stress vitamin' because of its importance to the proper functioning of the adrenal glands. (The adrenal glands are situated above the kidneys and secrete adrenaline and noradrenalin. See Chapter 7 for more information.)

A deficiency of pantothenic acid is often a factor influencing the inadequate production of these adrenal gland hormones. It also results in lowered resistance to infection. When volunteers were fed a pantothenic acid antagonist in combination with a diet low in the vitamin, they suffered from depression, fatigue, irritability, restlessness, muscle cramps, gastrointestinal upsets and poor muscle co-ordination. The symptoms disappeared when the vitamin was reintroduced into the diet.

Pantothenic acid is widely distributed in nature, occurring naturally in eggs, legumes, brewer's yeast, wheat bran and various whole grains.

The refining of wheat reduces its pantothenic acid by about fifty per cent.

## Biotin
Biotin, another member of the B-complex, is important for healthy nerves, bone marrow, cell growth, fatty acid production, the metabolism of carbohydrate, fat and protein and the utilization of other B-complex vitamins.

Deficiency signs and symptoms include leg cramps, depression, fatigue, insomnia and poor appetite.

Antagonists to this nutrient are alcohol, avidin (a substance in raw egg white), coffee and sulfa drugs. It is partially destroyed by cooking.

Natural food sources include eggs, legumes, brewer's yeast, sardines and whole grains.

## Inositol
Inositol is a compound that occurs in the brain, muscles, liver, kidneys and the lens of the eye. It works with other nutrients to produce lecithin.

This nutrient is yet another member of the B-complex. It helps to prevent hardening of the arteries, and it reduces cholesterol formation.

A deficiency of this nutrient may lead to arteriosclerosis ('hardening of the arteries'), high blood cholesterol, constipation and obesity. Alcohol and coffee are inositol antagonists.

Natural food sources include citrus fruits, milk, nuts, brewer's yeast and whole grains.

## Para-aminobenzoic Acid (PABA)
This is another member of the B-complex. It is important for blood cell formation, for the activity of intestinal flora, protein metabolism and healthy skin.

Deficiency signs and symptoms include constipation, depression, digestive disorders, headaches and nervousness. Alcohol, coffee and sulfa drugs are antagonistic to PABA.

Natural food sources of this nutrient include green leafy vegetables, nutritional yeast, wheatgerm and yogurt.

### Pangamic acid (vitamin $B_{15}$)

Pangamic acid aids the oxygenation of cells, respiration, the metabolism of protein, fat and sugar and the stimulation of the glandular and nervous systems.

Deficiency signs and symptoms include heart disease, nervous and glandular disorders and diminished cell oxygenation. Alcohol and coffee are antagonistic to this nutrient.

### Vitamin C (ascorbic acid)

Vitamin C contributes to the formation of *collagen*, a 'cement-like' substance that binds our cells together. We need vitamin C for various healing processes to take place and to reinforce our body's resistance to disease. Vitamin C is also important for the utilization of calcium, iron and folacin. If it is adequately supplied in the diet, it reduces our need for the B vitamins thiamin, riboflavin, niacin, pantothenic acid, pyridoxine and biotin by substituting for them and promoting their absorption.

The best vitamin C sources are found in foods of plant origin. Fruits highest in vitamin C are acerola (Caribbean cherry), apricots, blackberries, cantaloupe melons, cherries, elderberries, gooseberries, grapefruits, guavas, honeydew melons, kumquats, lemons, limes, oranges, papayas, red currants and strawberries. (An average serving of strawberries has about 88mg vitamin C.)

Vegetables (especially if eaten raw) highest in vitamin C content are asparagus, green beans, broccoli, Brussels sprouts, cabbage, carrots, cucumbers, leeks, parsley, red and green peppers, radishes, tomatoes and watercress. Green vegetables such as broccoli, Brussels sprouts, cabbage and kale have between 50 and 100mg of this vitamin per average serving. Potatoes, especially if cooked in the skins, are also a good source of this vitamin. Milk provides small amounts of vitamin C also.

*Smoking and vitamin C:* Studies done by the Canadian Government's Food and Drug Directorate show that cigarette smokers lose more vitamin C from their bodies than those who do not smoke. It appears that smoking increases not only vitamin C requirements, but also those of several other nutrients.

*The bioflavonoids (vitamin P):* Associated with vitamin C are a group of substances known as the bioflavonoids, or vitamin P, which occur in the pulp (but not the juice) of citrus fruits, especially in the white part inside the rind. They are also found in green peppers.

These substances appear to enhance the action of vitamin C in reducing inflammation and oedema and in promoting healing.

The bioflavonoids have proved useful to women suffering from menorrhagia (excessive menstrual flow) in that they have helped to relieve the condition. A group of French doctors have reported 'progressive improvement with the most marked improvement achieved by the third menstrual cycle' in treating women at one French hospital.

## The Fat Soluble Vitamins
Vitamins A, D, E, and K are soluble in fat. You therefore need to consume some fat in order to absorb them.

Whereas the water soluble vitamins not required are excreted in the urine, the fat soluble ones are stored in the body's fatty tissues. They can build up to toxic levels, so it's best to avoid taking these nutrients in supplement form. Use whole food sources instead.

### Vitamin A
Vitamin A has been implicated in PMS and difficult menstruation. Two South African researchers have reported that vitamin A has proven very effective in relieving

menorrhagia (heavy menstrual periods). This has been confirmed by practising doctors, among them Dr Jonathan V. Wright, as stated in an article appearing in the July 1983 issue of *Prevention*.

Vitamin A helps to build resistance to infection. It is important for fertility and for healthy mucous membranes (lining body cavities, e.g. the mouth and stomach). It is needed for healthy glands (e.g. the adrenals).

Symptoms of vitamin A deficiency include increased vulnerability to all kinds of infection and fatigue.

*Caution:* avoid vitamin A supplements. Excessive amounts of this nutrient can produce toxic symptoms such as yellowing and peeling of the skin, fragile bones and tissue damage.

Animal foods such as milk products, cheese and eggs provide vitamin A in ready-made form. Plant sources such as melons, apricots and carrots supply it in the form of carotene (also present in green leafy vegetables, although the colour is masked by the green pigment chlorophyll).

The best fruit sources of vitamin A are apricots, cantaloupe melons, cherries, papayas and peaches.

The best vegetable sources are beetroot tops, broccoli, carrots, endive (chicory), cress, dandelion greens, chicory (endive), kale, leafy varieties of lettuce, mustard greens, parsley, pumpkin, spinach, marrow (squash), Swiss chard, sweet potato, turnip greens and watercress.

### Vitamin D

Vitamin D facilitates the absorption and utilization of calcium and phosphorus. Until recently, it was believed that adults had adequate reserves of this vitamin in their tissues.

Our most reliable source of vitamin D is enriched milk, but butter, eggs, fish liver oils and milk contain small amounts, depending on the breed of the animals from which they are obtained and the amount taken in the diet.

Plant foods contain no vitamin D.

## Vitamin E

Vitamin E helps to oxygenate body tissues. It is a powerful anti-oxidant, and it contributes to a healthy blood circulation.

Vitamin E protects vitamin A, carotene and unsaturated fatty acids from oxidation in the body. High intakes of polyunsaturated fatty acids, found in vegetable oils, increase our need for vitamin E.

Ninety per cent of the active vitamin E (tocopherol) is lost when grains are refined and cereals are processed.

Our most valuable source of this nutrient is wheatgerm, which is removed during processing. Dependable sources of vitamin E are unrefined foods, especially green leafy vegetables, nuts, seeds and whole grains. It is important to store oils carefully to prevent rancidity, which destroys vitamin E.

The vitamin E content of fried foods is reduced by sixty-three to seventy-four per cent when they are frozen. Heating oils to high temperatures also reduces their vitamin E content.

## Vitamin K

Vitamin K, also known as the 'blood vitamin', helps the blood to clot readily, thus counteracting the tendency to excessive bleeding.

A varied diet of wholesome foods usually contains sufficient vitamin K for normal requirements. However, rich food sources include alfalfa sprouts, cow's milk, green leafy vegetables and unrefined vegetable oils, especially soyabean oil.

## Minerals

Minerals are essential constituents of all body cells and form the greater portion of the hard parts of the body such as bone, nails and teeth. They are important in maintaining our acid-base balance, as catalysts (helpers) in biological reactions and as regulators of muscle contractility and transmitters of nerve impulses.

The processing of foods significantly changes their mineral content in many cases. For example, many highly refined foods are high in salt, iodine and phosphorus and low in several other essential minerals. The most notable example of this is flour: seventy-five per cent of the iron, magnesium, potassium and zinc are lost in its refining, along with one hundred per cent of the calcium.

Nutritionists are growing increasingly concerned about the relationship between the mineral content of our food and optimum health.

Minerals are categorized as either macronutrient elements or micronutrient elements (trace minerals). The macronutrient elements are required in fairly large quantities by our bodies. They are calcium, chlorine, magnesium, phosphorus, potassium, sodium and sulphur. The trace minerals, needed only in small quantities, include chromium, cobalt, copper, fluoride, iodine, iron, manganese, selenium, silicion and zinc. The content of trace minerals in our food, particularly that of chromium, copper, iodine, selenium and zinc, is influenced by the soil in which the food is grown.

Of the macronutrients, magnesium and sodium have already been dealt with in Chapter 4.

## Calcium

Calcium is needed for the proper functioning of nervous tissue, normal clotting of blood and for the maintenance of sound bones and teeth. Emotional stress and prolonged periods of bedrest increase our calcium requirements; so do high protein and high fat diets.

Vitamin D supplies must be adequate for this mineral to be properly absorbed. Vitamin C and lactose (milk sugar) enhance calcium absorption.

High calcium foods include vegetables such as bok choy (pak choy, or uncurled green cabbage), broccoli, collard greens, dandelion greens, kale, legumes, mustard greens, turnip greens and watercress. Green leafy vegetables containing oxalic acid (e.g. spinach and chard) are good calcium sources, but the oxalic acid prevents proper absorption of the calcium. Citrus fruits and dried figs are high calcium foods, as are milk and milk products—cheese, milk (non-fat) and yogurt made with non-fat milk. Miscellaneous sources of calcium include blackstrap molasses, carob flour (the pulverized seed pod of a Mediterranean plant, which resembles cocoa) and soft fish bones.

## Chlorine

Chlorine, with potassium and sodium, is needed daily in quite large amounts. Together, these minerals determine the amount of fluid held in the body's tissues, and they attract nutrients from the intestines into the blood and from the blood into the cells. They are an essential part of glandular secretion. Chlorine also contributes to the formation of hydrochloric acid in the stomach.

It abounds in a wide variety of foods, including beetroot, carrots, celery, cheese, lentils, soya sauce and Swiss chard.

## Phosphorus

Phosphorus plays a major role in the maintenance of sound bones and teeth and in the regulation of the body's acid-base balance. It regulates energy release and helps in the absorption and transportation of nutrients.

The ratio of phosphorus to calcium in our diet is very important. Absorption of these nutrients is optimal when the ratio is one part phosphorus to one part calcium. This ratio has been upset by the increase in consumption of highly processed foods (e.g. commercially baked goods and soft drinks), which are high in phosphorus. With this increased intake, there has been a corresponding decrease in our consumption of milk, an excellent source of calcium. Fortunately, however, low phosphorus intakes rarely present a problem.

Excellent sources of this nutrient include dairy products and eggs.

## Potassium

Potassium, along with sodium, helps to maintain the electrical and chemical balance between tissue cells and the blood. These two nutrients must be in balance to maintain a normal flow of nerve signals and muscle contractions. Potassium, with sodium, is important for the maintenance of the acid-base balance of body fluids. It plays an important part in the release of energy from carbohydrates, proteins and fats. When the sodium level is high in relationship to the potassium level, health problems (e.g. migraine, muscle weakness, abdominal bloating and heart abnormalities) arise.

A potassium deficiency usually occurs not because of inadequate dietary intake, but because of diarrhoea, vomiting or the use of diuretics. A magnesium deficiency also makes it more difficult to retain potassium.

As with several other nutrients, foods in their natural state are highest in potassium, though never excessively high in sodium, as are many processed foods. Potassium is water soluble; it can easily be lost in the cooking water.

## Sulphur

Known as 'the beauty mineral', sulphur keeps the complexion clear and the hair glossy. It also plays a part in cell formation, respiration and in the synthesis of collagen, insulin and bile.

Natural food sources of sulphur include bran, Brussels sprouts, cabbage, kale and protein foods.

## Mineral antagonists

It is well to note that the following are antagonistic to the minerals described: contraceptive pills, too much coffee and tea, excessive stress, lack of exercise, habitual use of aluminium cookware (aluminium salts absorbed from) and excessive use of sugar, salt and alcohol.

## Cobalt

Cobalt forms part of vitamin $B_{12}$ (cobalamin), described earlier in this chapter. A deficiency may cause you to become tired easily. Good food sources of this nutrient include crab, oysters and sardines.

## Copper

Copper plays a role in many enzyme systems. It is essential for the production of ribonucleic acid (RNA), and is part of the nucleus of every body cell. It aids the proper functioning of the brain and nerves.

A copper deficiency contributes to decreased absorption of iron. It causes the life span of red blood cells to be shortened, and this leads to anaemia.

The richest source of copper is organ meats. Smaller amounts of this trace mineral are found in dry peas and beans, whole grain breads and cereals and green leafy vegetables grown in fertile soils. Like many other nutrients, copper is usually adequately provided if the diet consists largely of unrefined foods.

## Fluoride

This trace mineral is vital to well-being. It is also important for the maintenance of sound teeth and bones. A good source of fluoride is fish.

## Iodine

Iodine is needed by the thyroid gland (located in the neck) to make thyroxine, a hormone that regulates many body functions. A thyroxine deficiency could lead to a condition called goitre, which is still found in areas where the soil is iodine deficient.

Foods containing iodine include broccoli, cabbage, carrots, garlic, lettuce, onions and pineapple. Seafood and foods grown in iodine-rich seacoast soils are other good sources.

## Iron

Iron is a vital component of the red colouring matter of

blood (haemoglobin)—the part that transports oxygen to all body cells. An iron deficiency leads to anaemia.

The richest natural sources of iron among vegetables include—chard, greens (beetroot, dandelion, kale, mustard), green leafy vegetables such as leaf lettuce and spinach, legumes, parsley and seaweed. Fruit sources of iron are dried fruit, notably prunes and raisins, Sharon fruit (persimmon) and watermelon. Iron can also be found in grains and seeds such as buckwheat, cereals (whole grain), millet, oatmeal, rice bran, rye, sesame seeds and whole grains. Finally, miscellaneous sources of this mineral include blackstrap molasses, egg yolk, brewer's yeast, ocean perch, sardines and shellfish.

## Manganese

This trace mineral is needed to activate numerous enzymes and for the proper utilization of fats. A deficiency may lead to sterility.

Among the best sources of manganese are green leafy vegetables, nuts, unrefined breads and cereals grown on healthy soils, wheat bran and wheatgerm.

## Selenium

Selenium is needed for the maintenance of a good blood circulatory system, to reinforce the body's natural defence mechanism and for general well-being. It works with vitamin C and vitamin E to help detoxify the body. A selenium deficiency has been linked with high blood-pressure and premature ageing.

Good sources of this nutrient include asparagus, eggs, garlic, mushrooms, brewer's yeast, seafood and whole grains.

## Zinc

Zinc is essential for the synthesis of body protein and for the action of many enzymes. It also acts as a catalyst in many other biological reactions. It plays a role in carbohydrate metabolism, in that it is needed for insulin to work.

A diet high in phosphorus, such as that consumed by large numbers of people in civilized countries, interferes with zinc absorption. Up to eighty per cent of the zinc in whole grains is lost during the refining process. Also, women on contraceptive pills run the risk of developing a zinc deficiency. Among the zinc deficiency symptoms are loss of fertility, low resistance to infection, slow healing and poor appetite.

Green leafy vegetables, nuts and oysters are especially rich sources of this trace mineral.

## Complex Carbohydrates

Complex carbohydrates, or 'slowly digested' carbohydrates, consist of sugar, starches and dietary fibre. They are mainly found in such foods as wholewheat flour, brown rice, fresh corn and sugar cane. When these foods are refined, however, they lose a considerable quantity of valuable nutrients.

Formerly, starch was the most familiar of the complex carbohydrate group. Now, however, dietary fibre is gaining recognition.

### Dietary fibre

The fibrous part of plants is known as dietary fibre. It comprises cellulose and hemicelluloses, pectin and lignins. Most of these remain undigested in our system and serve chiefly as a source of bulk. Interestingly, dietary fibre prevents not only constipation, but also diarrhoea.

Perhaps the best source of dietary fibre is the outer layer, or bran, of whole grains. Unfortunately, the bran is removed during processing to produce the white flour and white rice consumed by so many individuals. In this respect, oats are the exception, for they are not subjected to the refining most other grains undergo. The rolled oats you purchase are the whole grains that have been rolled or cut into flakes, and it is this minimum of preparation that gives oats their nutritional superiority over most other breakfast cereals. Moreover, recent research indicates that the gums contained in oats add to their soluble dietary fibre, and are effective in reducing cholesterol levels in hypercholesterolemic patients (those with high blood cholesterol levels).

Other sources of dietary fibre include blackberries, raspberries, dates and black and butter (lima) beans.

## Fats (lipids)

A diet high in fats seems to increase prostaglandin production (refer to Chapter 2 for information on prostaglandins). This in turn is implicated in menstrual and premenstrual difficulties. As with caffeine (see section on caffeine, to follow), a mechanism may exist by which restriction of fat could bring about relief from unpleasant menstrual and premenstrual symptoms.

### Why use fat at all?

We need fats to help provide energy, to conserve heat and for the proper functioning of all body cells. We need fats for the production of sex hormones and other hormones and for important intestinal bacteria to thrive. We also require fats as carriers of the important fat soluble vitamins A, D, E and K.

Nutritionists have found that some persons suffering from oedeoma of the feet and legs have responded well to the addition of 30ml (2 tablespoons) salad oil to the diet. The American Heart Association, in fact, recommends the incorporation of 30 to 60ml vegetable oil to the daily diet to help keep the blood fat level within normal limits.

When fats are eaten, they are broken down during digestion into glycerin (glycerol) and fatty acids (sometimes referred to as vitamin F). Three of these fatty acids cannot be manufactured by the body and must be provided by the diet because they are essential to health (essential fatty acids, or EFAs). Some nutritionists believe that one of these, *linoleic acid*, is in fact vital. Good sources of linoleic acid include nuts, seeds, wheatgerm and the oils from these foods.

Unrefined vegetable oils are among the principal sources of EFAs. Polyunsatured fats, which help to reduce cholesterol build-up in the walls of arteries, are the best type of fat to consume. Safflower oil is the most polyunsaturated. Sunflower, soyabean, corn and sesame seed oils follow in descending order.

## Dangers of excessive fat intake

Having briefly explained why fats are important in the diet, it's time to mention that high fat intakes, particularly in the form of saturated fats (mainly of animal origin, e.g. butter, cream and meat) have been linked with various diseases, notably those affecting the blood circulatory system. As already mentioned, too, a high fat intake has been associated with increased prostaglandin production, which is thought to underlie certain menstrual and premenstrual problems.

With the higher consumption of convenience foods, the saturated fat intake of so-called civilized nations has increased dramatically; so have disorders linked with this dietary indiscretion. Today, the fat intake of many people in affluent countries contributes between forty and forty-five per cent of the total calorie intake. In Asia, by contrast, the fat consumed by most persons represents only between ten and twenty-five per cent of the total calorie intake.

To help you reduce your dietary fat intake to a healthful level, and so influence existing related problems, here are a couple of shopping and cooking tips. It is best to avoid buying oils or fats labelled 'vegetable', which usually means 'saturated'. Buy instead a specific type of oil, e.g. safflower or sunflower. Secondly, it is best to grill, steam or bake foods rather than fry them.

## Caffeine

Caffeine has been reported to increase prostaglandin production, thus aggravating the symptoms of dysmenorrhoea and its associated PMS. In Chapter 2, I explained what prostaglandins are and how they affect the uterus. I pointed out, too, some of the side-effects of the prostaglandin-inhibiting medications prescribed by many doctors.

Although prostaglandins have been implicated primarily in dysmenorrhoea, a recent double-blind study has shown a prostaglandin inhibitor (mefenamic acid, also mentioned in Chapter 2 page 22) to be effective relief for PMS symptoms. (A double-blind study is an investigation in which neither the subject under study nor the investigator working with the subject or data knows what the subject is receiving.)

It appears that a mechanism exists whereby restricting caffeine intake helps to alleviate difficult menstruation as well as premenstrual symptoms.

### Tea or coffee?

Coffee and tea (as well as cocoa and cola drinks) contain compounds collectively called *xanthines*. These substances include caffeine, theophylline and theobromine—powerful stimulants. They act on the nervous, respiratory (breathing) and cardiovascular (heart and blood vessels) systems. They increase the excretion of water from the body, along with important nutrients. Some side-effects of an excessive intake of xanthines are chronic insomnia, stomach upsets and persistent anxiety and depression.

It is noteworthy that some common medications (e.g. cold remedies) contain caffeine. Please check the labels of any medicines you're planning to purchase.

The weaker the coffee or tea you drink, the less the xanthine content. The caffeine content of a 250ml (about 8 ounces) cup of coffee varies from 30mg for instant coffee to 150mg for drip or filter coffee. Percolated coffee rates about midway between these in caffeine content. The same size cup of tea, brewed for one minute, contains about 25mg caffeine. If brewed for five minutes, the caffeine content increases to about 65mg. Many commercially-sold soft drinks contain between 30 and 50mg caffeine per 250ml (8 ounce) glass.

Decaffeinated coffee retains only about five per cent of caffeine. The safety of the chemicals used in the decaffeination process is, however, being questioned. Coffee substitutes are made from roasted, ground cereals. They contain no caffeine.

## Herbal teas
These contain no caffeine and their variety is almost endless. Brew them as you would regular tea, and sweeten them with a touch of honey, if you wish.

Camomile, peppermint, red raspberry and rosehip are among the most popular herbal teas.

## Carob powder
This cocoa and chocolate alternative is made from the ground seed pods of a Mediterranean tree and comes in the form of a powder resembling cocoa. It has a pleasant taste, somewhat sweeter than that of cocoa, and you can grow to like it quite easily.

Carob contains no caffeine, only two per cent fat (chocolate has fifty-two per cent) and does not inhibit the absorption of calcium, as do cocoa and chocolate. Moreover, those who are allergic to cocoa products are usually able to use carob with safety. Although carob powder contains no caffeine or other stimulant, it does contain some tannin which may disagree with persons sensitive to this ingredient.

## Alcohol
It has been found that one or two drinks actually decrease uterine contractions, which are thought responsible for some of the pain of dysmenorrhoea. Alcohol gives diameter to blood vessels and facilitates blood flow.

The bad news is that alcohol is antagonistic to several minerals and vitamins and is not recommended for use by those experiencing menstrual and premenstrual difficulties, except of course for a drink or two on occasion. Those suffering from hypoglycaemia should, of course, avoid alcoholic beverages altogether.

## Water

Nutritionists consider water to be the most important nutrient. It is the body's medium of transportation for many nutrients, it is a shock absorber, a temperature regulator and a lubricant. It serves to remove wastes from the system. Whereas even a cup of black coffee contains 5 calories, water contains absolutely none.

How much water should you drink daily? Your thirst will guide you. The body has its own thirst-regulating mechanism. It lets us know when we need to drink and how much.

### Bottled water

This may be spring water, purified tap water, distilled water or spring-type water.

Purified water is water from which minerals have been removed, while artificial spring water is distilled water to which minerals have been added. As with all foods, read the label carefully to know what's inside a bottle of water.

## Diet Plan for a Symptom-free Menstrual Cycle

— Drastically reduce sodium (salt) added to food during preparation and cooking and at the table.

— Curtail consumption of refined sugars.

— Decrease intake of saturated fats.

— Increase dietary fibre intake.

— Dramatically cut down on, or eliminate from the diet, over-processed (including convenience) foods. These foods are sadly devoid of many essential nutrients.

— Significantly increase your intake of fresh vegetables and fruits grown on healthy soils, to ensure a better supply of essential minerals, vitamins and other important nutrients.

— Store, prepare and cook all food to conserve, as much

as possible, the essential nutrients they contain.

— Omit, or drastically reduce, caffeine intake by substituting tea, coffee, cocoa and commercially sold soft drinks with water, unsweetened fruit juices, freshly pressed vegetable juices, herbal teas and milk.

— Eliminate, or significantly reduce, your consumption of alcoholic beverages. Alcohol is antagonistic to many vital nutrients.

— Make complex carbohydrates (as provided by whole grains, vegetables, nuts, seeds and other wholesome natural foods) a significant part of your diet.

— Eat adequately of protein foods, but be wary of high-protein diets which place extra demands on the body and increase the need for certain other nutrients.

— If you are troubled by symptoms of low blood sugar (hypoglycaemia), eat five or six small, wholesome meals, as opposed to three large meals, evenly spaced throughout the day. These meals should incorporate the principles outlined in this diet plan.

Finally, but not the least important, eat your meals in a relaxed, pleasant environment and eat them slowly.

# CHAPTER 6

# Exercises for Pain-free Periods

In Chapter 3, I mentioned the relationship between exercise and the body's own natural pain-relieving agents (endorphins). I pointed out that these natural analgesics are more readily available to people who exercise regularly than to those who do not.

Several studies have indicated a correlation between regular exercise and the relief of premenstrual tension, swelling of body tissues and abdominal cramps. Other studies have pointed to the poor performance of athletes during the four or so days before menstruation and on the first two days of the flow.

In their book entitled *It's Your Body*, Dr Niels Lauersen and Steven Whitney recommend that exercises be done a week before menstruation to strengthen the abdominal muscles and keep the body in better condition. They point out that dancers and athletic women have fewer menstrual complaints than less active women.

These specific problems aside, probably the greatest everyday value of regular exercise is the release of nervous tension. According to J. M. Ramsey (Professor of Biological Sciences at the University of Dayton in Ohio and author of *Basic Pathophysiology: Modern Stress and the Disease Process*), the entire muscular and hormonal systems are prepared either for the action of fight or flight during emotion. If there is no outlet for this emotion in the form of action, there is a progressive build-up of tension and possible maintenance of the elevated tension level for prolonged periods of time. Eventually, this state of tension favours the development of a number of stress-related disorders in some individuals. These disorders include recurrent headaches, insomnia, depression and problems connected with the stomach and intestines.

The specially selected exercises which follow have been designed to promote pelvic health in general, and to relieve difficulties (such as congestion) related to the menstrual cycle in particular. These exercises are all based on yoga principles, which have been in existence for centuries, and upon which many other highly effective forms of exercise are based. The training that women receive in preparation for childbirth, for example, is essentially based on yoga, regardless of the name given to the specific approach.

For more than a decade, I have taught these exercises to hundreds of women with a wide variety of problems. I present them to you unhesitatingly, confident that if you practise them faithfully when *not* menstruating, they will serve you well when you are, and in the difficult preceding days.

**Before You Begin**
The exercises to follow are safe and effective. As with any other exercise programme, however, *please check with your doctor* and obtain his or her approval before beginning. General rules for practice:
1. Practise regularly. The results you gain today are lost in forty-eight hours. Do your exercises daily, but if that is not possible, do them at least every other day when not menstruating. It is also wiser to practise for ten to fifteen minutes every day, or every other day, than one hour only once a week.

The author of *Yoga Simplified for Women* has stated that hysteria and neurasthenia (nervous debility), the nightmare of many a worried woman, could hardly find lodging in a body regularly and systematically trained each day by effective yoga exercises particularly suited to women.

2. Exercise at the same time each day or evening to establish the habit. The initial difficulty in doing so will soon pass if you remind yourself that it's an investment in better health and productivity.

3. Practise on an empty, or almost empty, stomach (not immediately after eating).

4. Empty your bladder and wear loose clothing so as to be comfortable and able to breathe freely.

5. Always do warm-up exercises to begin with, to avoid injury.

6. Practise on a padded surface (e.g. a carpeted floor). I shall refer to this surface from now on as the 'mat'.

7. *Never* hold your breath during the exercises. Synchronize your breathing with your body movements.

8. As you progress in your practice, maintain your completed position for a longer period of time, for it is through this 'holding period' that you derive the most benefits.

9. The exercises are presented in a certain sequence, but you can modify it to suit your particular needs. For maximum benefit, however, I suggest that you follow the Semi-reverse Exercise (Fig. 13) and the Spinal Stretch (Fig. 14) with the Pelvic Stretch (Fig. 10).

## Warm-ups

Just as a dancer warms up before a performance, a pianist plays scales and an athlete limbers up in preparation for a race, so too should you always warm up your body before an exercise session.

Warm-ups slightly increase body temperature, reduce stiffness, improve blood circulation and prevent pulls and strains.

Here are five superb warm-up exercises to get you started.

## The Butterfly

*How to do it*

1.   Sit naturally upright on your mat. Fold one leg inward; fold the other as well so that the soles of the feet are together.

2.   Grasp the feet with both hands and pull them toward you until they are as close as is comfortable (Fig. 3).

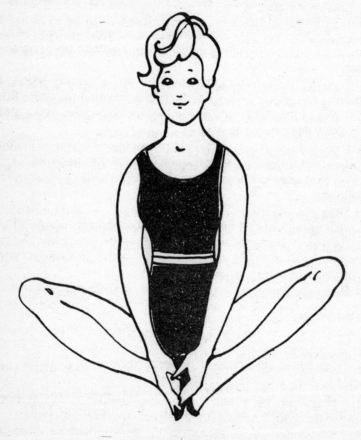

Fig. 3
Drawing of the Butterfly

3.   Still holding the feet securely, flap the knees down and up—like a butterfly's wings—several times in smooth succession. *Don't* hold your breath; keep breathing naturally.

4.   When you begin to tire, support yourself by placing your hands on the mat behind you, lean back slightly and stretch out the legs and rest.

*Notes:*

— I do about one hundred leg flaps in about one minute, almost every morning.

— The Butterfly is excellent for limbering up the ankle, knee and hip joints and for promoting good blood circulation to the lower pelvis.

— Instead of holding on to the feet, you may support yourself by putting your hands on the mat behind you, with fingers pointing away from you, and flap the knees down and up as in the basic warm-up.

I sometimes begin with this version and, as I lose my initial morning stiffness, proceed to the basic exercise.

— You may use this exercise, other than a warm-up, as follows:

Do steps 1 and 2 of the basic exercise.

Still holding on to the feet, press the knees as close to the mat as comfortable. Hold this knees-down position for a slow, silent count of six to begin with (longer as you progress). Remember to keep breathing normally.

Bring the knees up again. Stretch out the legs and rest.

## Ankle Rotation

*How to do it*

1.   Sit comfortably and naturally erect on your mat, with legs stretched out in front.

2.   Bend one leg at the knee, pass the corresponding arm under the bent knee to lift it off the mat and support it.

3.   Slowly and smoothly rotate the ankle clockwise three or four times (Fig. 4); rotate it counterclockwise the same number of times.

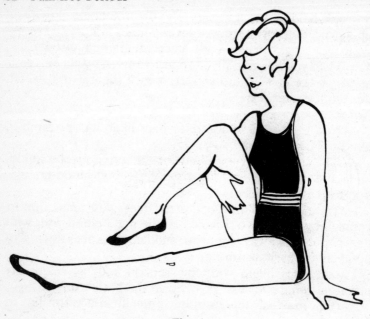

Fig. 4
Drawing of Ankle Rotation

4.   Rest the leg and repeat steps 2 and 3 with the other leg. Remember to breathe naturally throughout these warm-ups.
*Notes:*
   — Rotating the ankles is excellent for keeping the joints supple, for strengthening the feet and for promoting a good blood supply in the legs.
   — Keeping the circulation in the legs healthy helps to reduce congestion and discomfort.


### The Pelvic Tilt (on 'all fours')
*How to do it*
1.   Get on your hands and knees on your mat, like a table on four legs. Keep your body as level as possible. Check that you are breathing naturally.

2.  When next you *breathe out* (exhale), push your hips downward. At the same time, lower your head and straighten your arms. Your back should now assume a convex arch (Fig. 5).

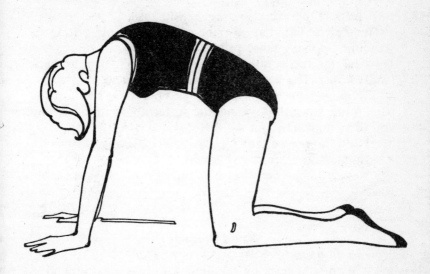

Fig. 5
Drawing of the Pelvic Tilt (on 'all fours')

3.  Exhalation complete, inhale and relax your body into the beginning position.
4.  Repeat steps 2 and 3 several times in smooth succession. Then rest.
*Notes:*

— Focus attention on moving your hips, rather than arching your shoulders, as you practise this warm-up.

— This exercise is excellent for keeping your pelvis freely movable, for strengthening the spine, and for easing backache.

— Pelvic tilting also tones and firms the abdominal muscles.

Practise the Pelvic Tilt as a non warm-up exercise, thus:
— Follow steps 1 and 2, described above.
— Maintain the convex arch of the back for a slow, silent count of six (longer as you become more adept).
— Inhale and relax.
— Repeat the exercise once, if you wish.

The Pelvic Tilt may also be practised lying, sitting or standing, applying these principles:

1.   Feel for the concave arch at the small of your back (waist level). The idea is to reduce or eliminate this arch.
2.   Remove your hands. *Exhale* and press the small of the back firmly toward or against the surface beneath or behind you (e.g. floor, chair or wall).
3.   Hold the pressure as long as your exhalation lasts.
4.   Inhale and relax your back.
5.   Repeats steps 2 to 4 several times in smooth succession. Rest.

### Knee Presses

*How to do them*
1.   Lie on your back on the mat, with legs outstretched.
2.   Bend one leg at the knee and as you exhale, bring the bent leg toward the chest. Hold it there for a slow count of three while breathing naturally (Fig. 6).

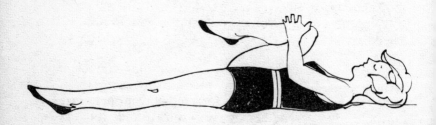

Fig. 6
Drawing of Knee Press

3.   Inhale, stretch out the leg and rest.
4.   Repeat steps 2 and 3 with the same leg three or four times.
5.   Repeat steps 2 and 3 the same number of times with the other leg. Rest.
*Notes:*
   — The Knee Presses help to strengthen the back muscles and relieve backache.
   — They help to dispel gas from the stomach and intestines.
   — They are excellent in helping to combat constipation.


## The Lying Twist

*How to do it*
1.   Lie on your back on the mat, with your legs outstretched and your hands under your head to make a 'pillow'. Keep your elbows pressed to the mat throughout the exercise to help to stabilize your shoulders.
2.   Bend your legs, one at a time, and bring the knees toward the chest. Legs are together.
3.   As you exhale, tilt the knees toward the mat on one side (Fig. 7). Inhale and bring the knees to the middle.

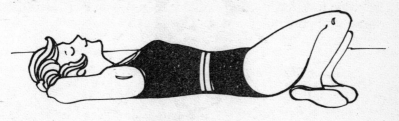

Fig. 7
Drawing of the Lying Twist

4.   Continue the exercise by tilting the knees to the mat on the *other side*. Inhale and bring the knees up to the middle again.

5.    Repeat steps 3 and 4 in slow, smooth succession several times, remembering to tilt the knees on the *exhalation*. Stretch out the legs and rest.

*Notes:*
   — The Lying Twist is superb for toning up the muscles of the abdomen and back.
   — It keeps the pelvis freely movable and improves pelvic circulation.
   — It helps to keep the midriff trim.

## The Exercises
### The Star

*How to do it*
1.    Sit naturally upright on your mat with legs stretched out in front.
2.    Fold one leg inward and position the heel in line with the knee of the opposite leg.
3.    Fold the other leg in the same way, placing the soles together.
4.    Clasp your hands around the feet *without shifting their position*.
5.    Exhaling, pull up on the toes and bend forward at the

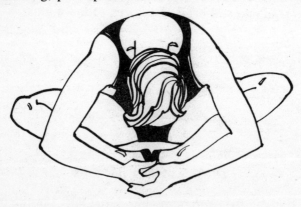

Fig. 8
Drawing of The Star

hip joints (*not* at the waist), aiming the face toward the feet.
6.   When you can bend no farther, relax in this position and keep breathing as you slowly and silently count to six (increase the count as you become more flexible). (Fig. 8)
7.   Inhale and slowly resume your beginning position. Rest.
    Repeat the exercise once, if you wish.
*Notes:*
    — This is an excellent exercise for toning and firming the inner thigh muscles and the perineum, and for improving the circulation to the lower pelvis.
    — It helps to keep the hip, knee and ankle joints flexible.
    — It is superb for keeping the spine flexible, and for relieving backache and back fatigue.
    — The Star contributes to improved digestion and better elimination.

## The Spread-leg Stretch

*How to do it*
1.   Sit naturally upright on your mat, with legs spread as far apart as comfortable. Place your hands on your legs, palms down.
2.   Exhale and bend forward at the hip joints (*not* at the waist—keep the torso erect), and slide your hands downward as if to touch the feet (Fig. 9).
3.   When you can bend no farther, hold your position (*do*

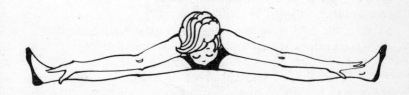

Fig. 9
Drawing of the Spread-leg Stretch

*not* hold your breath) for a slow, silent count of six to begin with (longer as you become more adept). Breathe naturally as you maintain the position.

4.   Inhale and slowly return to your beginning position. Rest.

Repeat this exercise once, if you wish.

*Notes:*

— The Spread-leg Stretch brings an excellent supply of blood to the perineal area (lowest part of the torso), thus contributing to the health of the pelvis.

— It tones and firms the inner thigh muscles and improves the circulation in the legs.

— It helps to keep the spine flexible and beneficially affects the myriad nerves branching off the spinal column.

— Diligent practice of this exercise will contribute to relief from menstrual cramps and backache.


## The Pelvic Stretch

*How to do it*

1.   Sit on your heels, Japanese style.

2.   Put your hands on the mat behind your feet, fingers pointing away from you.

3.   Inhale and *carefully* tilt your head slightly backward, press on your palms and raise your bottom off your heels as high as comfortable (Fig. 10).

4.   Maintain this position for a slow, silent count of six. Later, when you're practised, hold the position longer. Remember to keep breathing naturally.

5.   Inhale and resume your beginning position. Rest.

Repeat the exercise once, if you wish.

*Notes:*

— The Pelvic Stretch gives a delightful, therapeutic stretch to the upper thighs, groins and front of the torso and improves the blood circulation to this entire area.

— It strengthens the back.

— As you hold the position, the blood circulation to the

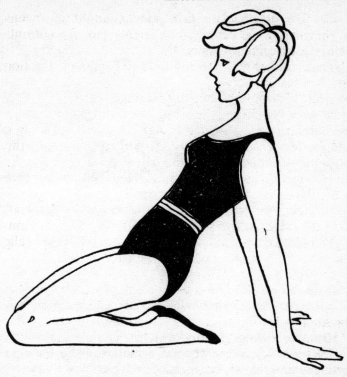

Fig. 10
Drawing of the Pelvic Stretch

pelvic area is facilitated, for the relief of existing congestion.

An excellent counter position to this exercise is the Curling Leaf (Fig. 12) which will be described later.

## The Pelvic Thrust

*How to do it*

1. Lie on your back with legs bent at the knees and the soles of the feet flat on the mat, a comfortable distance from your bottom. Position your arms alongside your body, palms down.

2.    Inhale, press down on the feet and arms and slowly raise first the hips, then the rest of the torso in one smoothly connected movement (Fig. 11).

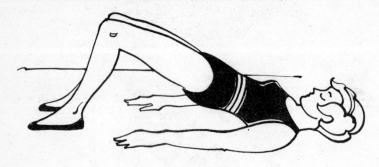

Fig. 11
Drawing of the Pelvic Thrust

3.    Hold this position for a silent count of six to begin with, and keep breathing evenly. (Later, you can maintain your completed position for as long as you can with ease.)
4.    Resume your beginning position, *in reverse*, lowering first the shoulderblades, then the middle of the back and finally the hips, slowly and smoothly. Stretch out your legs and rest.

You may repeat this exercise once.

*Notes:*
— The Pelvic Thrust strengthens the back and helps to relieve backache and back fatigue.
— It helps to relieve congestion in the pelvis.
— It tones and firms the abdominal muscles.

## The Curling Leaf

*How to do it*
1.    Sit on your heels, Japanese style.
2.    Bend forward and rest your forehead on the mat (separate your legs if necessary).

3.  Rest your arms beside you, palms upturned (Fig. 12).

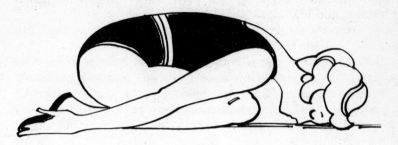

Fig. 12
Drawing of the Curling Leaf

4.  Stay in this position for as long as you're comfortable, breathing naturally.
5.  Return to your beginning position slowly.
*Notes:*
— The Curling Leaf is excellent for relaxing the back.
— As you breathe in and out while in this position, the gentle pressure of the thighs on the abdomen effects a beneficial massage to abdominal structures. This is useful in helping to prevent constipation.
— This exercise encourages a healthful blood supply to the upper body.
— Feel free to turn your head to the side if you can't breathe properly in the position described above.

### The Semi-reverse Exercise
*Caution:* if you have heart or lung disease, high blood-pressure or hiatus hernia (hernia of the respiratory diaphragm), do *check with your doctor* before attempting this exercise.
*Do not* practise the Semi-reverse exercise during the menstrual flow or if you're experiencing 'vacuum head-aches'.

*How to do it*

1.   Lie on your back with your arms beside you, palms down, and legs stretched out in front.

2.   Bend your knees and position your feet comfortably close to your bottom.

3.   Straighten your legs upward, one at a time. Press your hands and elbows firmly against the mat and kick backward to raise the hips. Keep your elbows on the mat, but support your hips with your hands, thumbs in front (Fig. 13).

4.   Maintain this position for a slow, silent count of six

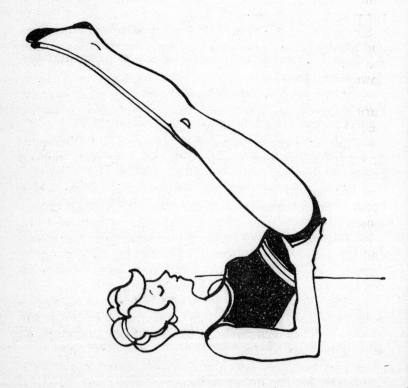

Fig. 13
Drawing of the Semi-reverse Exercise

(longer as you become more comfortable doing this exercise).

5.   To come out of the position, keep your head firm on the mat (slightly tilt the chin upward if necessary), put your arms beside you and *slowly and carefully* lower your torso, from top to bottom, in a smoothly connected manner. When your hips are down, stretch out your legs and rest.

Repeat the exercise once, if you wish.

*Notes:*

— If you are overweight, you may use a prop, such as a wall or the edge of a sturdy piece of furniture, to help you get your hips off the mat.

Simply put your feet on the prop, press down on the arms and hands and push the hips upward. Once the hips are off the mat, support them with the hands and kick the feet upward and backward. Ask a friend to help.

— Although it is inadvisable to practise this exercise during menstruation, you can safely do the Legs Up exercise (see Fig. 18).

— The Semi-reverse exercise gives a delightful therapeutic stretch to the back muscles and helps eliminate built-up tension.

— The contraction of the abdominal muscles, which occurs during the practice of this exercise, helps to restore muscle tone and eliminate fat stored in the abdominal walls.

— The organs within the trunk are revitalized: stomach and intestines, liver, pancreas, spleen, bladder and reproductive organs. This brings about an improvement in digestive, metabolic and endocrine processes.

— The thyroid gland, located in the neck, receives a better blood supply and its function is improved. Since the thyroid gland influences the body's metabolic processes, all cells and tissues benefit.

— This head-low hips-high position is one of the most favourable for facilitating drainage of the blood vessels of the lower body, particularly those of the abdominal and pelvic organs. It is, therefore, of immeasurable value in easing congestion of these parts.

## The Spinal Stretch

*Caution:* do not practise the Spinal Stretch during the first few days of menstruation. Do not practise it if you have a prolapsed uterus or a hernia.

*How to do it*

1.   Begin as for the Semi-reverse exercise, just described. Bend the legs and rest the soles flat on the mat.
2.   Bring the knees to the chest.
3.   Straighten the legs so that the feet point upward.
4.   Kick backward with both feet at once until the hips are raised. Keep the arms on the mat.
5.   Push the feet backward and continue doing so until they touch, or come close to touching, the mat behind you (Fig. 14). Stop when you have reached your comfortable limit.

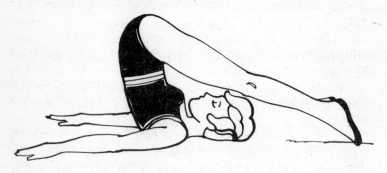

Fig. 14
Drawing of the Spinal Stretch

6.   Hold this position for a slow, silent count of six (longer as you become practised). Breathe naturally.
7.   To come out of position, *slowly and carefully* roll your spine, in a smooth and connected manner, onto the mat, until the hips are down. If you press your arms firmly to the mat, it will help you do this without strain. Keep your head on the mat.

Bend your knees; lower your feet to the mat, stretch out and rest.

*Notes:*

— This exercise, done properly, can stretch the spine nearly fifteen per cent above the normal, from the back of the head to the tip of the spine. In so doing, it takes pressure off the many nerves branching off the spine. It improves the circulation in the spinal cord. Indirectly, it brings about improvement in the internal organs influenced by these nerves.

— The stretching of the back muscles contributes to their elasticity and tone. This helps to strengthen the back and reduce backache.

— Because of the head-low hips-high posture assumed during this exercise, pressure within the abdomen and pelvis is eased, and the organs within them function better.

— Muscles and ligaments supporting the uterus and ovaries are strengthened.

— Practised faithfully, this is an excellent exercise to combat constipation, obesity, sexual debility and rigidity of the spine.

— Don't worry if your feet don't touch the mat behind you right away. As the spine loses its initial stiffness, they will.

— You may place a prop (a pile of cushions, a low stool or a box) behind you so that your toes do touch something. This will serve as a guide to your progress toward touching the mat itself.

## The Spinal Twist

*How to do it*

1. Sit on the mat with your legs stretched out in front of you.
2. Bend the *left* leg at the knee and place the *left* foot beside the *outer* aspect of the *right* knee.
3. Smoothly swivel your upper body to the *left* and place both hands on the mat at your *left* side. Turn your head and look over your *left* shoulder (Fig. 15).

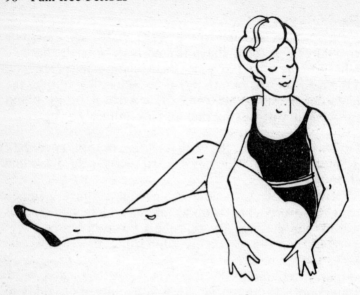

Fig. 15
Drawing of the Spinal Twist

4.   Hold this position for a slow, silent count of six (longer as you become more practised), breathing as naturally as possible.
5.   Carefully untwist and resume your beginning position.
6.   Repeat steps 2 to 5 in the opposite direction (substitute the word 'left' for 'right', and vice versa, in the instructions).
*Notes:*
— This is possibly the best exercise for providing safe torsion (twisting) of the spine. This spinal rotation provides a stimulating massage to myriad nerve roots branching off the spinal cord. The structures supplied by these nerves also benefit.
— The lower back muscles receive a therapeutic stretch which helps to preserve their tone and minimize backache.
— The kidneys benefit and elimination of wastes is improved.

— The adrenal glands (located above the kidneys) are revitalized. According to Dr Steven Brena, to revitalize these glands is to improve the whole circulatory system and 're-charge' energy in the 'electric batteries' of our body cells.

## The Modified Sit-up

*How to do it*

1. Lie on your mat with your legs stretched out in front and your arms beside you.

2. Bend the legs and slide the heels slowly toward you. *As soon as* the feet are flat on the mat, stop. The idea is to have the feet not too close to the bottom.

3. Place the hands on the thighs, palms down.

4. Exhaling, *carefully and slowly* tilt your chin toward your chest as you raise your upper body. Your hands will begin to slide toward the knees.

5. Keep coming up slowly, reaching for the knees, but not necessarily to touch them. Keep your eyes riveted on the fingers.

6. When you feel your abdominal muscles become as tight as you can comfortably tolerate, hold your position (Fig. 16). *Do not* hold your breath.

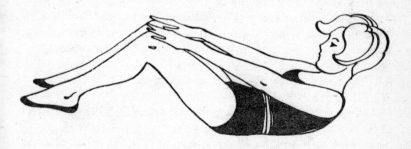

Fig. 16
Drawing of the Modified Sit-up

7.   Maintain your sit-up for a slow, silent count of six (longer as your back and abdomen become stronger).

8.   Inhale and slowly return to your beginning position, in reverse. Rest.

Repeat this exercise once, if you wish.

*Notes:*

— This modified sit-up will *not* strain your back. It will protect and strengthen it.

— As you maintain the sit-up in synchronization with breathing, your abdominal and pelvic organs will receive a natural massage that will improve the circulation to them.

— The abdominal muscles will be toned and firmed, lending more effective support to the organs in the abdomen and pelvis.

— Practise this marvellous exercise during television commercials, on the beach or in the park (if you can do so comfortably and unobtrusively).


## Squatting

*How to do it*

1.   Stand with your feet comfortably apart.

2.   Slowly bend your knees and lower your body, as if to sit on your heels. You may stretch out your arms in front to help you keep your balance.

3.   When your bottom is as close to your heels as you can manage, hold your position for a slow, silent count of six (longer as you become more comfortable with the exercise). Relax your arms and hands (Fig. 17).

4.   Come out of position, in reverse and rest.

*Notes:*

— You may hold on to a stable prop (e.g. a table or sturdy chair) to help you get into the squatting position.

— Regularly practise ankle rotation (Fig. 4) to keep your ankles supple. You need flexible ankles to squat properly.

— Look for ways of incorporating squatting into your daily schedule. Squat to dust low furniture, to weed the

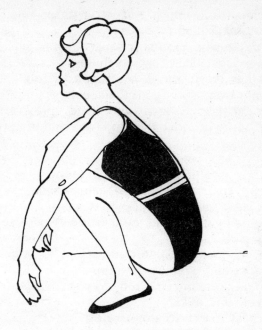

Fig. 17
Drawing of the Squatting position

garden, to chat informally on the beach or in the park. I squat in the bathtub to shampoo my hair with a spray attached to a hose.

*Benefits of squatting:*

— Squatting is the most natural position for defaecation (emptying the bowel).

— Squatting helps to make the perineum more elastic, and therefore a better support for the pelvic organs.

— It reduces the curve of the spine at the small of the back. Consequently, the muscles and ligaments supporting the spine are relieved and there is less pressure on the discs between the bones making up the spine. As a result, the back is strengthened and relaxed, and back discomforts are reduced.

— Squatting tones and strengthens the abdominal muscles, ankles and feet.

— People who habitually squat seem to suffer less from varicose veins, piles (haemorrhoids) and prolapse of the uterus than those who don't. If you already have varicose veins, however, *don't* hold the squatting position for long. Instead, alternately squat and stand up, several times in succession, to improve the blood circulation in the legs.

## The Perineal Exercise

'Perineal' refers to the perineum which, as mentioned earlier, is the lowest part of your torso. It's the area between the external genitals and the anus (back passage).

*How to do it*

1.   Sit, lie or stand comfortably. Breathe naturally.
2.   *Exhale* and tighten your perineum.
3.   Hold the tightness as long as your exhalation lasts.
4.   Inhale and relax.
5.   Repeat steps 2 to 4 once. Rest.
6.   Repeat the entire exercise several times throughout the day.

*Notes:*

— Here are some places where you can do this exercise: on the bus, in the car while waiting for a red light to change to green, at boring parties and meetings—any place where you feel comfortable doing it. No one will know that you're exercising.

— This is a time-proven exercise that's a 'must' for any woman interested in maintaining good pelvic health. It strengthens and tones the perineum, which helps to support the pelvic organs. It contributes to more intense sexual pleasure. It combats 'stress incontinence of urine', that is, the tendency for urine to trickle from the bladder, involuntarily, when you cough, sneeze or run.

### Legs Up

The Legs Up exercise is excellent for relieving that dragging-down feeling often experienced before menstruation and on the first and second days of the flow.

It helps to reduce swelling in the feet and counteract fatigue. By elevating the legs, the return blood flow to the heart is aided because the valves of the large blood vessels, which prevent back flow, are given a rest.

*How to do it*

1. Lie on your mat near a wall and rest your feet against the wall. Your legs slope, forming about a forty-five degree angle with the wall (Fig. 18).

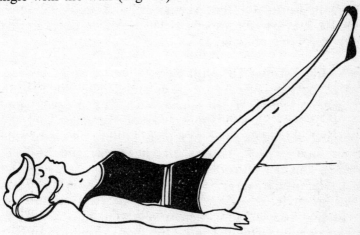

Fig. 18
Drawing of the Legs Up exercise

Don't be concerned if you can't achieve the exact position. The general idea is to position your legs so that they are as high as you can manage with absolute comfort.

2. Rest your arms and hands quietly beside you. Close your eyes and focus your attention on your breathing. Breathe slowly, smoothly and rhythmically.

3.   Each time you inhale, visualize filling your whole system with refreshment and renewed energy. Each time you exhale, visualize breathing fatigue away from your legs and feet and indeed from your whole body.

4.   Stay with your legs up for at least three minutes to begin with. Increase the time as you become increasingly comfortable in this position.

To come out of position, bend your legs and pull your knees toward your chest, roll onto your side and use your hands to help you up.

*Note:*

Whereas the Semi-reverse posture is not recommended during menstruation, this exercise can and should be done. Practise it every day, especially when you've done a great deal of walking or standing.

## Reducing Fatigue Through Good Posture and Carriage

Correct posture and carriage are essential to optimum health of body and mind. Watch someone who is depressed. Note the somewhat sunken appearance of the chest and the drooping shoulders. The stooping posture places undue strain on the back muscles and ligaments and leads to fatigue. This can, and often does, develop into backache and back pain, which aggravate an existing depression and create a vicious circle.

Holding yourself tall when sitting, standing or walking enhances mental equilibrium. If the shoulders droop and the upper back is rounded, strain is placed on the spinal muscles. The resulting back strain progresses to backache and later to pain. These generate depression, again a vicious circle.

You cannot separate the physical from the emotional. Many of the aches, pains and muscle spasms we experience are because we sit, stand, lie and work with bodies improperly aligned. All these health problems have psychological components—they generate anxiety, frustration and depression.

Habitual slouching and other faulty postures cramp internal structures and adversely affect blood circulation. The lungs do not expand fully and oxygen intake, necessary for the health of every cell, is insufficient for optimum well-being. The consequences of such postures include fatigue, lack of energy, and eventually nervous exhaustion; also related are various discomforts, aches and pains. Concentration is adversely affected and so is the ability to make decisions and to act rationally.

There is yet another condition related to incorrect posture, although the relationship is often unsuspected. It is called *enteroptosis*. It means that the stomach, intestines, liver, pelvic organs, and sometimes the kidneys, are literally dragged down and remain in a position that's incompatible with optimum functioning. When these structures do not function as they should, a whole host of symptoms appear and undermine our good health.

Improper posture and carriage retard the blood circulation, causing the blood in the abdomen and pelvis to stagnate. This contributes to constipation through a general 'self-poisoning' process.

### Posture related to emotional states

There is an intimate relationship between how you feel physically and how you feel emotionally. If you stand elegantly, your muscles send a message to your brain to say that you feel marvellous and in control. If, however, you stand downcast, with shoulders drooping and head bowed, the message relayed to the brain is a negative one suggesting stress.

### Occupational postures

Many of us develop 'occupational postures' because of the nature of our work. For example, surgeons may acquire round backs because of the way they often have to stand during surgery. Dentists may become high-shouldered on one side because they have to accomodate themselves to a confined space. Hairdressers may bulge at the abdomen because of certain stances they must adopt habitually, and fashion models may find themselves developing rigid backs because of the carriage they're required to assume as they display their clothes.

## The secret of good posture

The secret of acquiring and maintaining good posture is to take measures to counteract these occupational attitudes we may have to adopt temporarily. For instance, if you are hunched over a work table for an hour assembling the intricate parts of some piece of equipment, take several minutes break periodically to offset that posture. Sit or stand naturally erect and squeeze the shoulderblades together. Stand and stretch from top to toe, perhaps bending backward slightly while tightening the seat muscles and inhaling deeply. Carefully make circles with your head, clockwise and counterclockwise, to keep the neck flexible and to prevent tension build-up.

## The key to good posture

The key to good posture is the control of the pelvis. The pelvis connects the torso to the legs. A review of Chapter 1 will confirm that it is formed by two large (innominate) bones, with part of the spine wedged between them (sacrum and coccyx). The pelvis provides a base for the spine, and it is supported chiefly by back, abdominal and seat (buttock) muscles.

To help with the pelvic control so important to correct alignment of the spine and for good posture, please practise the Pelvic Tilt regularly. It was described earlier in this chapter (see Fig. 5 for the 'all fours' position, page 83), and you can do it in any of four positions.

Whether you sit or stand, lie down or get up, bend, reach, lift or carry, your key to good posture is maintenance of the normal curves of the spine. Any position, gesture, action or movement that alters these curves will place strain on spinal structures, weaken them, produce discomfort and make the back more vulnerable to injury.

To maintain normal spinal curves, you must keep your back and abdominal muscles in good tone and avoid being overweight. Efficient muscles are essential to the support of the spine and consequently to good posture. It is not only sedentary workers who need to exercise. Those whose occupations entail physical labour may be using certain muscles habitually, to the neglect of others that are equally important to the health of the torso. Regular, suitable exercise will help to stretch shortened muscles that cause postural imbalances. It will help to keep joints freely movable and less vulnerable to injury. The exercises presented in this chapter will meet these requirements. Remember to *check with your doctor* and ask if they are suitable for you or compatible with any treatment you are receiving.

For quick reference, here are the exercises you need to do daily (or every other day), when not menstruating, to promote and maintain good back and abdominal muscles and for a healthy spine:

### For the back
— The Pelvic Tilt in any of the four positions (see Fig. 5 for the 'all fours' position, page 83)
— The Knee Press (Fig. 6, page 84)
— The Star (Fig. 8, page 86)
— The Pelvic Thrust (Fig. 11, page 90)
— The Curling Leaf (Fig. 12, page 91)
— The Semi-reverse Exercise (Fig. 13, page 92)
— The Spinal Stretch (Fig. 14, page 94)
— The Spinal Twist (Fig. 15, page 96)
— Squatting (Fig. 17, page 99)

## For the abdomen
— The Pelvic Tilt in any of
the four positions
— The Pelvic Stretch (Fig.
10, page 89)
— The Pelvic Thrust (Fig.
11, page 90)
— The Modified Sit-up (Fig.
16, page 97)
— The Semi-reverse
Exercise (Fig. 13, page
92)

# CHAPTER 7

# Reducing Stress

## Stress and the Menstrual Cycle

The menstrual cycle is very sensitive to changes in emotional states. In London, during World War II, gynaecologists observed and documented an amazing number of cases of amenorrhoea (non-appearance of menstrual periods). As the women reporting this absence of menstruation lost their anxieties and relaxed, their periods returned.

Similarly, women who travel a great deal or undergo major changes in lifestyle (e.g. a separation or divorce, a new job or the death of a family member) tend to miss periods. I remember missing mine when I left home for the first time to travel overseas to England to study nursing. As I adapted to my new surroundings and shed some tensions, my periods returned as spontaneously as they had disappeared.

As pointed out in the section on magnesium (see page 50), several symptoms asociated with difficult menstruation are similar to those people under stress experience. When you understand the physiological (pertaining to body function) and psychological (referring to the mind) changes that occur in response to stress, you will better comprehend the relationship between stress and various health disorders.

To help you gain this understanding, here's a synopsis of what stress is and what takes place when you're faced with a stressful situation.

## What is Stress?

Stress may be viewed as *external* ('something out there') such as work or competition. It may also be regarded as *internal*, such as an individual's response to a challenge or threat (when she feels 'stressed').

The currently accepted view of stress is that it is a *transaction between the individual and the environment* (my emphasis) or, as suggested by R. S. Lazarus, it consists of demands that tax or exceed our personal resources. The late Hans Selye, acknowledged as perhaps the most outstanding expert on stress, defined it as the non-specific reaction of any organism to the demands made on it.

Every individual defines and creates stress in her own terms and deals with it in a very personal way. Some of us, because of our distinctive lifestyles and personal values, experience stress more acutely than others.

### Sources of stress

Failure, frustration, conflict, uncertainty and anxiety are among the most harmful forms of stress, or *distress*. Pleasant forms of stress, or *eustress* (to use Dr Selye's coined word), include a passionate kiss and a reunion with friends or relatives after a long separation.

What determines the difference between these is *the way we view events and how we cope with them*. The most common and deleterious form of stress is what is referred to as 'hassle', that is, the small conflicts that simmer and sometimes boil over during our day to day dealings with children, spouses, lovers, bosses and colleagues. I can cite many of these encountered during my part-time work in a hospital setting. Because hassle is insidious and cumulative, and because it is not always visible, it is all the more destructive to health.

## Changes Occurring During Stress

Laboratory studies show that body hormone and enzyme levels alter during stress. They change to help us combat stress. More than thirty different hormones are involved. By measuring their concentration, researchers can assess the intensity of the stress.

In any acute stress situation (e.g. preparing to avoid a head-on motor vehicle collision), these chemicals 'burn themselves off' after the incident. With an ongoing stress, however (e.g. 'hassle'), the chemicals accumulate in our system and wreak havoc with our health.

The following are some changes that take place in our body when we are under stress. Even though we may not see or feel them, they are occurring nevertheless.

— Blood circulation speeds up. The coronary arteries (supplying heart muscle) dilate, or widen. Pulse rate increases. Blood-pressure rises. Blood cells are drawn from storage and minerals from bones. Peripheral (at the extremities) blood vessels constrict, or tighten. Blood clotting time shortens.

— More sugar enters the bloodstream. Proteins are withdrawn from lymph glands and converted into sugar. *Salt is retained in abnormal amounts*.

— Digestion is temporarily impaired. Appetite loss occurs.

— Muscles of the neck and back become rigid, braced for 'fight or flight'.

— Hair may 'stand on end'.

— Breathing rate increases.

The foregoing, and other symptoms, occur because stress hormones are activated. Among these are:

— ACTH (adreno-cortico-trophic hormone), secreted by the pituitary gland (hypohysis) in the brain.

— Adrenalin and noradrenalin (epinephrine and nore-pinephrine), collectively known as the 'catecholamines', secreted by the medulla (middle; plural medullae) of the adrenal glands located above the kidneys.

— Corticoids secreted by the cortex (shell, or outer part) of the adrenals.

— CRF, a hormone produced by nerve cells.

Briefly, in times of 'fight or flight', when there is need for self-protection either through confrontation or retreat in their diverse forms, nervous impulses activate CRF, which stimulates the pituitary to produce ACTH. In turn, ACTH rouses the manufacture of corticoids, while other nerve stimuli cause the medullae of the adrenal glands to secrete their hormones. When the various hormones enter the bloodstream, the changes described take place.

It is noteworthy that the pituitary is the 'master gland', the 'conductor of the endocrine orchestra'. It influences the function of every other endocrine gland in the body, which of course includes the ovaries. The ovaries, you will recall (see Chapter 1), are intimately involved in the menstrual cycle.

## Coping With Stress

Coping embraces all the devices we use to neutralize threats to our stability and enable us to function effectively.

How we appraise both external and internal stressors (agents producing stress) is *whether or not we feel in control*. We are less liable to experience acute stress if we know, for instance, that a stressful situation won't last long or that we are fairly resilient.

One coping strategy you may wish to try consists of using *direct action*. Change the situation, retreat promptly or relinquish a goal. Direct action means *changing one's relationship with the environment* (or, as R. S. Lazarus would put it, changing one's commerce with the environment). We can't always use direct action, though. We may have to resort to *palliative* (comfort) *measures*. These include denial (not thinking about it), intellectualization (taking a philosophical stance), detachment ('it has nothing to do with me') and self-deception.

*These methods don't make the threat or challenge go away, but they sometimes help us to feel better temporarily.* They give us a period of respite, during which we can replenish our energies and regain perspective.

Successful coping, therefore, does not always involve active mastery over our environment. In some circumstances, retreat, tolerance, compromise or disengagement may be the healthiest possible response.

*Practical hints*

Here, now, are some practical tips to apply to help you cope better with various distresses and increase your control over 'external' circumstances.

— Know, first of all, that mental, physical and emotional health are inextricably linked.

— When you're ill or uncomfortable, examine your attitudes toward the illness or discomfort. Are they negative or positive? Study those around you who seem to cope well. Try to learn what they do or did to help resolve difficulties. Can you profit from their example? Can you look at your problem as a stepping stone toward growth?

— Try to avoid great swings in levels of activity, whether at work or play. Aim for evenness of pace.

— Daily observe yourself, to become more attuned to your body and sensitive to its cues. No machine, however sophisticated, can do this for you the way you yourself can. A twenty-minute period spent daily in relaxation or meditation will train you for this (techniques are given later in this chapter).

— Determine your goals. Don't permit anyone to set these for you. This also applies to choosing your occupation. According to Hans Selye, even if you make a bad choice of spouse, don't make a bad choice of job because it's likely to be where you spend most of your time and energies.

— Learn to say 'no', graciously but guiltlessly. Say 'no' to the company of those who deplete your energy reserves and who depress you. Say 'no' to being pressured into making a decision when you're not physically or mentally at your best, (e.g. when experiencing the symptoms of PMS or dysmenorrhoea). Decline invitations to socialize when you know in your heart that you should spend that time in solitude, to recharge your energies and repair your health. Be charming but firm when you say 'no'. There's no need for explanations either, unless you want to make them.

— Express, rather than suppress, your feelings. Resentments locked inside you fester and ultimately hurt you more than the ones against whom you hold them.

— Find healthful outlets for pent-up emotions: write down your feelings, even if you have to tear up the paper afterwards. I've experienced tremendous relief on the occasions on which I've done this. Clean out a few cupboards, play tennis, take a brisk walk—you may not be able to walk away from your troubles, but you can certainly walk off some of the force of their initial impact. I've proven this many times.

— Schedule appointments to coincide with the days you are symptom-free, if you know when these days are likely to be. Try not to make important decisions or sign contracts on the days when you don't feel well. If there's an examination forthcoming, be sure to get enough sleep and relaxation in the preceding twenty-four hours.

— Spend some time on yourself each day. You devote so much to your work, family and friends. How much time do you give to yourself? One guilt-free hour a day will do much to preserve or enhance your integrity. During this hour, do whatever you enjoy most—a long, leisurely soak in the bathtub, window shopping, reading poetry, painting or meditating.

— Resist the 'superperson' urge. Keep your surroundings neat, but not sterile. Accept yourself with your shortcomings and you will find it easier to accept others with their frailties. You will get along better with others, and this in turn will enhance your feeling of well-being.

— Learn to laugh. Laughter is one of the best tension breakers there is. Sometimes, learn to laugh at your problems. You may realize that they are not as insurmountable as you may have thought.

— Above all, love and respect yourself. Try to develop a good sense of self-worth. Psychologists say that a poor self-image is a form of self-rejection, which invokes a great deal of distress.

## Breathing as a Stress-reducing Technique

The breath is perhaps our handiest, most effective natural tool for combating stress. We carry it with us wherever we go, it's not usually noticeable or distracting to others, and it's not burdensome as a rule. And yet, we all but forget its existence until we have some respiratory (breathing) difficulty, such as blocked nasal passages, nasal congestion, asthma or a common cold.

The air we breathe in contributes to the process of providing nourishment to all cells, the brain cells included. Our breath is influenced by our state of mind, and vice versa. During life's moments of 'fight or flight', breathing tends to become rapid and irregular in response to hormonal changes. If we consciously regulate our breathing—slowing it down and making it more rhythmical—it will effect beneficial changes in our emotional climate. It's virtually impossible to be hysterical or to panic when breathing slowly and evenly and focusing attention on the breathing process.

Tests have shown that, after a prolonged period of breathing in a controlled manner, the electrical resistance of the skin is raised. The *Electrical Skin Resistance Test* is one of the most sensitive methods by which to demonstrate the activity of the sympathetic nervous system. A raised electrical resistance of the skin occurs during calm mental states.

Research indicates that breath control techniques designed to relax muscles and mind will also deeply relax internal structures as well (e.g. heart, stomach, intestines, glands) without producing drowsiness or sleep.

### Diaphragmatic breathing

A good place to start in using your breath as a stress

relieving device is to re-learn diaphragmatic breathing, which you did naturally as an infant but likely lost the art of doing as you grew up.

This type of breathing brings into play the muscle separating your chest cavity from your abdominal cavity (the diaphragm). It provides the following benefits:

— it helps to lower high blood-pressure to within normal limits.

— it counteracts anxiety states, promoting calm and control.

— it improves blood circulation and venous return of blood to the heart (which helps to reduce the heart's work load).

— it improves the functioning of several internal structures through a natural, gentle massage action.

— it aids the digestion of food.

— it aids the elimination of wastes from the system. It is a natural anti-constipation remedy.

— it helps to soothe and calm the nerves.

— it helps you to look less worried, more relaxed and more youthful.

You may breathe diaphragmatically in almost any position— sitting, standing, lying on your back or even upside down! But it's virtually impossible *not* to breathe this way when lying prone (face downward).

*How to do it*

1.  Lie prone, with your face turned to one side and your arms positioned for comfort (Fig. 19). Close your eyes and relax as totally as you can.

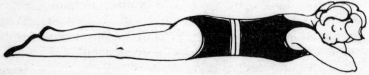

Fig. 19
Drawing of Diaphragmatic Breathing in the prone position

2.   Inhale slowly, smoothly and as deeply as possible *without strain*. As you do so, imagine, or visualize, breathing right down into your abdomen, filling the top, middle and bottom of your lungs. Be aware of your abdomen making closer contact with the mat (or surface on which you are lying).

3.   Equally slowly and smoothly, exhale completely and feel your abdominal muscles relax. Visualize emptying your lungs thoroughly.

4.   Exhalation complete, repeat steps 2 and 3, several times in smooth succession.

5.   Continue this rhythmical, diaphragmatic breathing for a minute or two to begin with, increasing the time as you become more practised.

For maximum benefit, practise diaphragmatic breathing several times daily, whether menstruating or not.

## The Mountain Breath

This breathing exercise permits better ventilation of the lungs and promotes the nourishment of all body cells. Its overall benefits are the same as those derived from regular practice of diaphragmatic breathing.

You may do it standing, applying the same principles given for the sitting version that follows. Practise daily.

*How to do it*

1.   Sit naturally erect on a low stool, or on a mat in a folded leg position ('tailor fashion'). Close your eyes if you wish.

2.   Position the hands as if in prayer, palms together and fingers pointing upward.

3.   Inhale slowly, smoothly and deeply *without strain*, simultaneously raising the arms until they are fully stretched overhead (palms are still together). (See Fig. 20, page 116.) Visualize filling the top, middle and very bottom of the lungs to ventilate fully every bit of lung tissue.

4.   Inhalation complete, proceed without pause to exhale slowly, smoothly and thoroughly as you lower the arms to

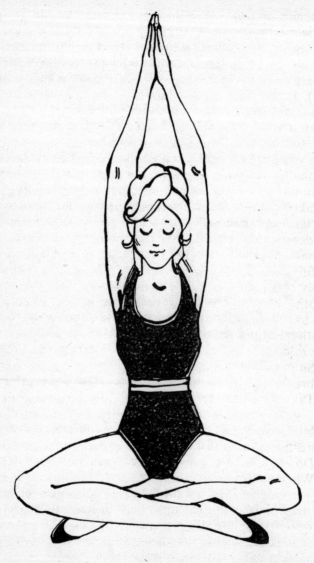

Fig. 20
Drawing of the Mountain Breath

the beginning position. Visualize emptying the top, middle and deepest recesses of the lungs completely.

5.   Repeat steps 3 and 4 several times in smooth succession. As you become more comfortable with this exercise, increase the number of respirations (inhalations and exhalations). Relax your arms and legs and rest.


## The Sighing Breath

Have you ever observed a child who has fallen asleep after an unhappy episode? Have you not noticed how, as pent-up emotion is spent and the child begins to relax totally, he or she takes a series of short, quick, jerky inward breaths and then lets out the inspired air in one long breath reminiscent of a deep sigh?

I have found the breathing exercise which follows very helpful on occasions when I'm too tense or upset to breathe deeply and evenly. At such times, I know that a few slow, smooth, deep breaths would calm me, but my chest is too tight to permit full lung expansion. So I practise the Sighing Breath instead.

*How to do it*

1.   Sit comforably and naturally upright. (You can also do this breathing exercise standing or lying.)

2.   Take a series of short inward breaths, instead of one long, slow one. It's like breaking up the one prolonged inhalation into several smaller ones—several successive inward sniffs—until you feel your chest expand and lungs fill. *Do not strain*.

3.   When you have filled your lungs, let out the air through your mouth in one smooth stream, as if cooling a hot beverage. *Alternatively*, you may exhale through your nostrils in the same steady manner.

4.   Repeat steps 2 and 3, as many times in succession as necessary (until you begin to relax and feel more in control). Resume regular breathing.

Practise the Sighing Breath whenever you are upset,

anxious or pressured. Practise it anywhere appropriate.

## The Alternate Nostril Breath

*Introduction*
One of the most distressing symptoms experienced by many women, premenstrually as well as during menstruation, is a 'vacuum headache'. This is the term that Dr Katharina Dalton gives to the type of headache which is due to the swelling of cells at the entrance of the nasal sinuses. This swelling blocks the nasal passages so that stale air accumulated inside cannot be readily expelled.

*Symptoms of vacuum headache*
Breathing becomes difficult. There is tenderness or a feeling of pressure over the eyes and cheek bones, corresponding to the location of the sinuses. This can develop into pain which may last from one day to seven days; bending down aggravates the pain.

*Allopathic remedies*
'Allopathic' is a word of Greek origin and means 'other than the disease'. Allopathic remedies, then, refer to drugs or treatments having no consistent or logical relationship to presenting symptoms. They are usually what doctors prescribe.

The usual allopathic treatment for vacuum headaches is restriction of fluid intake, diuretics to reduce oedema, nasal decongestants to relieve nasal congestion and analgesics to ease pain. These medications, however, if used long enough, often produce adverse effects that are just as troublesome as, or more of a problem than, the original symptoms for which the sufferer sought help in the first place.

*The nasal lining and menstrual cramps*
Turn your attention to the nose for a moment. Underneath the mucous membrane lining it there is another, thicker,

spongy tissue which can quickly fill with blood. This is 'erectile' tissue, found only in a few areas of the body: the genitals, the breasts and lining of the nose.

When this tissue engorges with fluid, it becomes erect. There is a close relationship between the nose and the other areas where erectile tissue is found. Ear, nose and throat specialists are, in fact, familiar with the 'honeymoon nose' experienced by newly-weds during the period of continual sexual stimulation.

It has been found that menstrual cramps are not infrequently related to an inflammation and discoloration of the lining in certain parts of the nose. When these areas are anaesthetized (rendered insensitive to pain) with a local anaesthetic, menstrual pains disappear. In fact, for some time in Germany, menstrual pain was effectively treated by cauterizing (burning) nerve endings in selected areas of the nasal lining.

## Alternation of the breath

There is more, however, to the swelling and shrinking of nasal erectile tissue. There is actually a regular, predictable pattern of alternate swelling and shrinking. When the air flow through one nostril is restricted through swelling, the other nostril is more open, so that air flow is predominantly through one or the other. In health, this right-left dimension of breath flow is predictable and regular, alternating roughly every hour and forty-five minutes to two hours.

In disturbed emotional states and other deviations from good health, this rhythm is altered. It changes, too, with irregular schedules of eating and sleeping and with infection and exposure to pollution. These observations, which have been well documented by research laboratories in the West and East, come under the heading 'infradian rhythm'. We are inclined to regard this phenomenon as recently discovered, but serious yoga practitioners have known of its existence centuries ago. It is in accord with the latest findings on 'right brain/left brain'.

## Benefits of alternate nostril breathing

To help restore regularity, rhythm and balance to this natural alternation of breath through right and left nostrils—and through it mental equilibrium and improved health—the Alternate Nostril Breath is perhaps unsurpassed. This breathing exercise will:

— help to relax body and mind;
— promote concentration and clear thinking;
— help to keep blood-pressure within normal limits;
— be a good antidote to insomnia; and
— can be used to relieve acute pain, e.g. headache.

## Preparing for the Alternate Nostril Breath

First, you must become familiar with diaphragmatic breathing (described earlier in this chapter). When you can breathe diaphragmatically in a slow, smooth and easy manner, you are ready for alternate nostril breathing.

*How to do it*

1.   Sit naturally upright, with head, neck and the rest of the spine in good alignment. Close your eyes. Rest your *left* hand in your lap. You'll use your *right thumb* to close off your right nostril when it's time, and *right ring finger* to close off the left nostril when necessary (Fig. 21).

2.   *Exhale* steadily through the nostril that is less blocked, closing the opposite nostril with the appropriate finger or thumb.

3.   *Inhale* steadily through the same nostril. Inhalation complete, release closure of the opposite nostril and close off the nostril through which you have just inhaled. *Exhale* through the open nostril.

4.   *Inhale* through the same nostril.

5.   Repeat steps 2 to 4 twice more (a total of six breaths through each nostril—one 'round').

6.   Relax your hand and take three normal respirations (inhalations plus exhalations).

7.   Do two more rounds of alternate nostril breathing, as outlined in steps 2 to 5.

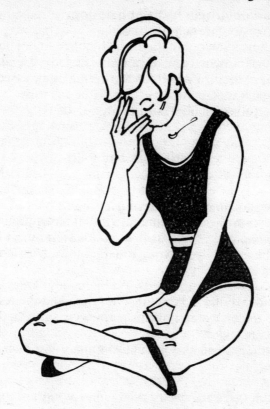

Fig. 21
Drawing: The Alternate Nostril Breath

Here, for your convenience, is an example of the sequence, beginning with the *left* nostril.
1.  Sit comfortably. Be as relaxed as possible. Close your eyes.
2.  *Exhale* ('out') through *left* (nostril).
3.  *Inhale* ('in') through *left* (nostril). *Out* through *right*.
4.  *In* through *right*.
5.  Repeat steps 2 to 4 twice more to complete one round.
6.  Relax your hand and take three normal respirations.

7.   Do two more rounds of alternate nostril breathing (steps 2 to 5). Resume normal breathing.

*Notes:*

— Breathe slowly, gently, noiselessly and *without strain*.

— Fully concentrate both on the breathing process and on the alternate opening and closure of the nostrils.

— Practise alternate nostril breathing daily.

## Breathing Away Pain

*How to do it*

1.   Sit or lie as comfortably as possible. Make sure your spine is well supported. Let yourself go as limp as you can and close your eyes. You may tie a dark scarf around your eyes to completely shut out light and hasten relaxation.

2.   Wilfully slow down your breathing. Make it smoother and more even.

3.   Rest your fingertips lightly on the painful area and take a long, steady inward breath. As you do so, visualize a soothing jet of water flowing along your arm and hands toward your fingers.

4.   Breathe out steadily, visualizing the water issuing from the fingertips, entering the affected spot and washing away the pain.

5.   Repeat steps 3 and 4 as many times as needed to bring a measure of relief.

6.   Relax your arms and hands and rest.

*How it works*

How is it possible to use breathing exercises to lessen pain? Those of you who have attended childbirth preparation classes will already be familiar with the use of different levels of breathing to correspond with various intensities of uterine contraction. You will remember how you decreased the depth of your breath and speeded up its rate as the contractions grew stronger; how you increased the depth and slowed down the rate as the contractions subsided. For those of you not acquainted with such breath control methods, here's how you can use respiration to quell pain or discomfort:

— Focus your whole attention on the breathing process so as to divert your thinking from the pain. By so doing, your former negative response to it will diminish.

— Consciously slow down the rate of respiration and try to make the breathing more even. As you do this, your mind will respond by becoming calmer; your blood circulation will improve so that the painful area will receive a better blood supply to help promote healing; your blood-pressure will become more stable; your heartbeat (and pulse) will slow down to help promote relaxation.

In exercises like the Alternate Nostril Breath, your attention is riveted not only on the breathing pattern and process, but also on the closure and opening of alternate nostrils. With the mind focused on these, awareness of pain is lessened.

## How to Relax Completely

In Chapter 3 (page 33) I referred to Dr Edmund Jacobson's observations on the value of relaxation in managing pain. Deep relaxation breaks the fear-tension-pain cycle and makes it easier to cope with the distress.

*Benefits of deep relaxation*

Relaxation training has been used with admirable success in a number of areas, e.g. childbirth, competitive sports, to help lower high blood-pressure and in the treatment of phobias (abnormal fears). Psychotherapists frequently train clients in the art of deep relaxation, which they say is antagonistic to anxiety.

Deep relaxation brings to the surface muscular and nervous tensions, the existence of which you may not even suspect. At this level, you are then able to release them voluntarily, in a conscious way. In doing so, you will be able to restore and maintain the natural harmony between body and mind which typify integrity and good health.

When you habitually practise deep relaxation, beneficial

changes occur in the functioning of all the body's systems, not only during practice, but also long afterwards. Some of these benefits include:

— a calmer mental state, more poise;

— better emotional balance, a more even temper, more control;

— improved concentration, better productivity;

— blood-pressure lowered to within normal limits;

— more youthful good looks.

## Best technique

The technique most commonly used is generally referred to as 'progressive' or 'progressive deep muscle' relaxation, and here is the version preferred by most of the hundreds of students I've instructed in it for at least the past ten years.

It's a good idea, when first attempting this technique, to ask a helper to read the instructions aloud so you can get the details right. You can also read them aloud into a tape recorder for future listening and practice. Spend between twenty and thirty minutes on this exercise and practise it *every day*.

## Basic relaxation positions

Lie supine (face upward) on the mat. Legs are outstretched in front and about 30cm (12 inches) apart to prevent tension building up in the thighs. Arms are well away from the sides of the body to avoid tension accumulating in the shoulders. Ideally, palms should be upturned. Shoulders are pulled down from the ears. The chin is tilted neither up nor down,

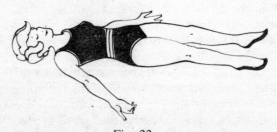

Fig. 22
Drawing: Deep Relaxation in the supine position

the head is well positioned. The eyes are closed (Fig. 22).

If you have a lower back problem and find the above position less than totally comfortable, you may modify it thus: bend your knees and place the feet flat, comfortably far from the bottom and about 30cm (12 inches) apart. Lean one knee against the other to discourage tension build-up in the thighs.

You may also practise this relaxation technique in a recliner (easy-chair). Simply modify the supine position, making sure that your neck, back, arms and legs are well supported and the body well aligned.

*How to do it*

1. Breathe naturally and let yourself sink into your mat or chair, with no resistance whatever. Periodically check to make sure that you're breathing regularly. *Do not* hold your breath at any time.

2. Direct your attention to your feet. Pull your toes toward you and push your heels away. Your legs will stiffen. Maintain (hold) the stiffness for a few seconds. Note how tight the legs and feet feel.

3. Now completely let go of the tightness. Relax the toes, feet and ankle joints. Note how limp and heavy they feel now.

4. Next, focus your attention only on your knee joints. Tighten, or lock, them. The legs will again stiffen. Hold the stiffness for several seconds and note the tension in the legs.

5. Totally release that tension. Unlock the knee joints, let go of tightness in the calves and thighs and let the legs go limp and heavy.

6. Turn your thoughts next to the buttock muscles. Squeeze them together as tightly as you can. Hold the tightness for a few seconds.

7. Release the tightness from the buttocks. Totally relax the hips.

8. Direct your attention to the small of the back (waist level). *Exhaling*, press it against or toward the surface on which you are lying. Hold the pressure for a few seconds— until your exhalation ends.

9.   Inhale, let go of the pressure and allow your lower back muscles to relax totally. (If necessary, repeat steps 8 and 9 until your lower back feels very comfortable and completely free of tension.)

10.   Turn your thoughts now to the upper back and focus attention only on the shoulderblades. *Inhale* deeply and squeeze them together, holding the squeeze as long as the inhalation lasts.

11.   *Exhale* and release the squeeze, completely relaxing the upper back.

12.   Pull the tips of your shoulders toward your ears. Hold the shrug for a few seconds.

13.   Relax the shoulders.

14.   Next, turn your attention to the front of your body, concentrating on the abdominal muscles. *Exhaling*, tighten the abdomen as fully as you can. Hold the tightness as long as your exhalation lasts.

15.   *Inhale* and relax the abdomen. Spend a few moments visualizing the contents of the abdominal cavity—intestines, glands, blood vessels. Visualize them relaxing and functioning more healthfully.

16.   Focus attention on the chest next. *Inhale* slowly, smoothly and deeply, *without strain*. Note how the chest expands as the lungs fill completely. Feel the chest muscles stretch.

17.   *Exhaling* steadily, relax the chest. Spend a few moments visualizing the contents of the chest cavity—lungs, heart, glands, blood vessels. Visualize them relaxing and functioning more healthfully. Also check your breathing to make sure that your respirations are gentle and even.

18.   Direct your thoughts next to the arms and hands. Tighten them. Raise the stiffened arms off their support as you *inhale*.

19.   *Exhale* and let the arms and hand collapse onto their support. Let go of tightness in the fingers and hands. Relax the forearms and upper arms. Check that the shoulders are still relaxed.

20. Roll your head from side to side a few times to mobilize tensions accumulated in the neck.

21. Re-position your head. Tilt your chin upward to stretch the throat gently. Hold the stretch for a few seconds.

22. Relax the throat. Relax your tongue.

23. *Carefully* raise your head slightly, tilting it forward as though to look at your chest. Feel the muscles at the back of the neck stretch.

24. Re-position your head and completely relax your neck.

25. *Exhaling,* open your jaws widely. Stick your tongue out as far as possible without hurting yourself. Open your eyes. Stare fiercely. Tense all your facial muscles.

26. *Inhale* and relax all your facial muscles. Close your eyes. Let go of tightness in your jaws, lips and tongue. Relax your cheeks, eyes and eyelids. Relax your brow. Visualize all fatigue draining from your face. Visualize your features becoming more composed.

27. Spend a few moments meditating on the soothing flow of your breath. With each inhalation, visualize your system filling with positive things, new energy and new hope. With each exhalation, visualize an outpouring from the system of everything negative and unwanted.

28. Allow your entire body weight to sink onto its support, confident that the support will safely bear it. Let yourself go completely. Don't hold back. Relax.

*Coming out of deep relaxation*

You will sense when it's time to resume your activities. But don't jump up suddenly. Give the body and mind time to adjust.

Open your eyes. Blink a few times if you wish.

Move the smaller parts of your body—wiggle your toes and fingers and rotate your wrists and ankles. If you feel like turning your head from side to side, do so. Tune into your body and follow its cues.

Stretch your limbs in a leisurely fashion. Take time to savour each delicious moment. Yawn if you feel the urge to do so. Carefully get up. Stretch from top to toe. Return to your schedule with renewed vigour and optimism.

## Meditation
Some people are suspicious of the word 'meditation'. It conjures up images of eastern mystics sitting as if in a trance, cross-legged on the floor. Others regard it as a ritual performed by, and suited only to, those belonging to religious sects. Neither impression is correct.

### What is meditation?
Simply, meditation is a technique used to quiet a restless mind and to dissuade it from dwelling on a thought or idea. It's a natural device used to relax the conscious mind without obliterating awareness. Doctors call this state 'restful alertness'.

### Meditation for stress-related disorders
Much of the fatigue and many of the nagging discomforts and ailments we experience are born of accumulated tension. Today's living provides never-ending stimuli for activating the 'fight or flight' mechanism inherent in all of us. It offers relatively few socially acceptable opportunities, though, for the actual fight or flight. The result of this is unresolved tensions that can generate conditions such as high blood-pressure, heart disease, migraine type headaches, gastrointestinal upsets and a host of nervous disorders. Enlightened doctors realizing this are recommending that their clients seek means of learning to cope naturally with such tensions, rather than rely wholly on drugs.

### The benefits of meditation
Regular meditation helps to dissolve and remove deep-rooted nervous strains. Researchers say that not even deep sleep or the dream state can eliminate such stresses as completely as meditation can. With the stresses removed, the meditator becomes more at ease with herself and with

others, more confident and more productive. She often finds that things which were formerly very upsetting begin to lose their impact and appear at least manageable.

## What produces the benefits?
During meditation, a unique state occurs. Oxygen consumption and carbon dioxide elimination decrease markedly without an alteration in their balance. This means that the blood circulatory system is functioning as it should. The heart's work load is lessened. Heart and breathing rates slow down, indicating a state of deep relaxation. Skin resistance increases significantly, which denotes a calm emotional state. The body's metabolic rate drops by about twenty per cent, with a corresponding lowering of blood-pressure. Lactate ion concentration in the blood, suspected to affect muscle tone adversely, as well as influence emotional states, decreases by about thirty-three per cent. Brain wave recordings (electroencephalograph, or EEG) show an unusual abundance of alpha waves, which implies that the brain is alert yet wonderfully rested.

## Preparing for meditation
Here are some essentials to observe before attempting to meditate, no matter what technique you plan to use.
— You must be able to sit quietly and keep relaxed for several minutes in order to meditate successfully. I suggest, therefore, that you become conversant with the deep relaxation technique, described earlier in this chapter.
— Always meditate before a meal so that the digestive processes do not interfere with concentration.
— Select a quiet place where you are unlikely to be disturbed.
— Sit comfortably, with the spine well aligned and supported if necessary. Rest your hands quietly in your lap or on your knees or on the arm-rest of a chair. Close your eyes. Spend a minute or two relaxing as completely as you can. Pay particular attention to your eyes, jaws and hands.

— Now focus your attention on your breathing. Breathe slowly, smoothly, evenly and noiselessly. Do not manipulate the breath in any way; simply let it flow naturally.

*How to meditate*
1.  Inhale steadily through the nostrils.
2.  Exhaling steadily through the nostrils, mentally say the word 'one'. (Alternatives to 'one' are 'peace', 'relax', 'calm' or any other pre-selected word that will not trigger a train of thought. You could also use a short phrase such as 'love and light'.)
3.  Exhalation complete, repeat steps 1 and 2, in smooth succession for five to twenty minutes.

If your mind strays from the breathing and repetition of your chosen word or phrase, gently guide it back. Be patient. It takes time, discipline and practice to keep your attention only on your meditation, but it's worth the effort.

As with deep relaxation, outlined earlier, make the transition from sitting quietly to resuming activity slow and smooth.

*Coming out of meditation*
1.  Open your eyes. Blink a few times if you wish.
2.  Stretch out your legs. Move about or massage any part of your body that seems to need it.
3.  Take a few slow, deep breaths.
4.  Slowly get up and stretch your body from top to toe.

*When to meditate*
Meditate at least once a day. Begin with five minutes, and work up to twenty minutes per session. Eventually, try to meditate for twenty minutes twice daily.

Meditate before a public appearance, an interview, a board meeting, an examination or before the children come home from school—any time you're anticipating a demanding situation.

Meditation is nature's tranquilliser—the cheapest and best there is.

# CHAPTER 8

# Herbs that Help

According to the late Dr Paavo Airola, herbs have been used as healing agents by every race on the earth since time began. As recently as the 1800s, no less than eighty per cent of medications available to physicians were derived from plants.

Today, herbs are employed as remedial agents in many parts of the world. In countries such as Africa, Central America, China, Mexico, the Pacific Islands and South America, herbs are widely used. In other countries, scientists are conducting research into many old-time herbal remedies after having ignored them for years. Take *Rauwolfia* (snakeroot) for example. It is the source of many modern sedatives and agents to lower high blood-pressure. *Digitalis purpurea* (purple foxglove) has provided a commonly used heart medication for ages. The Chinese ephedra (*Ephedra sinica*) is a natural source of ephedrine, a stimulant and relaxant of bronchial smooth muscle, still much used as a treatment for asthma. And *Sarsaparilla* root is being used to manufacture a male sex hormone tablet (testosterone) by a leading pharmaceutical company. In fact, most of the drugs currently prescribed by doctors come from plants or are synthetic variants of compounds originally found in plants; these include antibiotics which are obtained from moulds. It is estimated that the number of plant-derived drugs now used is about seventy per cent of the total.

In the USA, several reputable organizations are earnestly

seeking out plant remedies for a growing list of disorders because chemical drugs have failed. Among these conditions are arthritis, cancer, heart disease and multiple sclerosis (MS).

Some doctors argue that with plants, you can't know exactly what dose you're getting. Dr Andrew Weil, author of *Health and Healing*, who has had much experience with medicinal plants, points out however that whole plants have certain built-in safety mechanisms that are lost when certain elements are refined out of them, as in manufactured drugs. In other words, you can always tell if you're taking too much of a herb and you can then reduce the quantity or stop taking it.

## Herbal emmenagogues

Several herbs have what is known as an *emmenagogue* action, that is, they facilitate menstruation. Some have a direct effect on the reproductive tract, and others alter menstrual function by influencing the general state of health. Information on more than two dozen such herbs is given later.

## Preparing herbs for use

In preparing leaves, blossoms and small plants for use, it is best to make a herbal tea, technically known as an *infusion*. (This is not to be confused with a *decoction*, in which hard material such as barks, roots and seeds are boiled for a considerable length of time.)

*To make an infusion:*

To make an infusion, the usual proportions are 5ml (1 teaspoon) dried herbs to 250ml (1 cup) boiling water, or 28g (1 ounce) dried herbs to 600ml (1 pint) boiling water.

Place the herbs in a ceramic (never metal) container and pour freshly boiled water over them. Cover the container and let the herbs steep for about fifteen minutes. Stir the mixture, let it settle, strain it and let it cool to the desired temperature (it's best not to drink a very hot infusion).

Sweeten the tea with a little natural honey if you wish.

Always make a fresh supply of herbal tea when required.

*To make a decoction:*

Put 28g (1 ounce) bark, roots or seeds in a non-aluminium utensil with 90ml (1½ pints) water. Cover the utensil (or partially cover it) and let the mixture boil for thirty minutes. Turn off the heat.

Let the decoction steep for another 30 minutes. Strain and cool it. Drink one cupful. Store the rest in the refrigerator in a glass jar with a tight fitting lid. It will keep for about a week.


*Tinctures*

The medicinal properties of some herbs are destroyed by heat. Others will not yield their active ingredients to water. Some herbal extracts are therefore made with the help of certain types of alcohol. These are known as *tinctures*.


## Herbs Facilitating Menstruation (herbal emmenagogues)
### Amaranth (Amaranthum blitum)

Uses: To relieve menorrhagia (excessive bleeding during the menstrual period), either in the number of days or the amount of blood or both.

Dosage of fluid extract: ½ to 1 drachm (1.8-3.6ml).

As a decoction: Take a wineglassful three or four times a day.


### Anemone pulsatilla

Synonyms: Pasque or Easter flower.

Part used: Whole herb.

Uses: Nerve tonic, antispasmodic (agent that relieves spasm), diaphoretic (agent that increases perspiration) and for the relief of headache. Relieves feeling of fullness in the pelvis and weakness in the lower back.

Dosage of fluid extract: Five drops in a little water three times a day.

## Angelica
Synonyms: Garden angelica and Masterwort.
Parts used: Root, seeds and herb (usually the herb).
Uses: Diuretic. Excellent for suppressed and delayed menstruation.
Dosage: A wineglassful of the infusion about three times daily.

## Arrach (Chenopodium olidum)
Synonyms: Dog's Arrach, Goat's Arrach, Stinking Arrach, Stinking Goosefoot and Motherwort.
Part used: Herb.
Uses: For nervous troubles connected with female ailments. It has antispasmodic properties and facilitates menstruation.
Dosage: A wineglassful of the infusion three or four times a day.

## Balm (Melissa officinalis)
Synonyms: Sweet Balm, Lemon Balm, Cure-All and Honey Plant.
Balm is an abbreviation of Balsam, the chief of sweet smelling oils.
Part used: Herb.
Uses: Carminative (agent that expels gas), diaphoretic and febrifuge (agent that reduces fever). Excellent for delayed menstruation, to relieve pain before and during the periods and for suppressed menses (monthly flow).
Dosage: A wineglassful of the infusion three times daily.

## Basil, Sweet (Ocymum basilium)
Synonyms: Garden Basil and Basil.
Part used: Herb.
Uses: To relieve pain caused by delayed menses.
Dosage: A wineglassful of the infused herb three or four times daily.

**Black Cohosh (Cimicifuga racemosa)**
Synonyms: Black Snake Root, Rattle Root, Squaw Root and Bugbane.
Part used: Root.
Uses: Diuretic and emmenagogue. Excellent to help relieve pain in the back, pelvis and thighs. Good for suppressed menses and to regulate the periods.
Dosage: Ten to fifteen drops of the fluid extract in water three times a day for two or three weeks.

**Blue Cohosh (Caulophyllum thalictroides)**
Synonyms: Blue Berry, Squaw Root, Papoose Root, Blue Ginseng and Yellow Ginseng.
Part used: Root.
Uses: To regulate menstruation, as an antispasmodic and diuretic. Has been successfully used to relieve uterine inflammation.
Dosage: A wineglassful of infusion or decoction three or four times a day.

**Buchu (Barosma betulina)**
Synonyms: Bucku and Bancha Leaf.
Part used: Leaves.
Uses: To ease various menstrual discomforts and to relieve cystitis (inflammation of the bladder).
Dosage: A wineglassful of infusion three or four times a day.

**Catmint (Nepeta cataria)**
Synonyms: Catnep or Nep.
Parts used: Leaves and herb.
Uses: As an emmenagogue, antispasmodic, sleep inducer, relaxant and to relieve headaches.
Dosage: As an emmenagogue, it is preferable to use Catnep, not as a warm tea, but to express the juice of the garden herb and take it in tablespoon doses three times a day.

### Ephedra (Ephedra vulgaris)
Synonyms: Ephedrine, Epitonin, Ma Huang.
Uses: Remarkable effect on unstriped muscle fibres (as found in the uterus). It relieves swelling and acts as an antispasmodic.
Dosage: ½ to 1 grain of the tablet (30-60mg).

### Evening Primrose (Enothera biennis)
Synonym: Tree Primrose.
Parts used: Bark, leaves.
Uses: Sedative, to relieve gastrointestinal upsets and to alleviate various female complaints, such as pelvic fullness.
Dosage: From 5 to 30 grains (300mg to 2g).

### Fennel (Foeniculum vulgare)
Synonyms: Fenkel, Sweet Fennel and Wild Fennel.
Parts used: Seeds, leaves, roots.
Uses: To regulate the menstrual periods and as a carminative.
Dosage: A wineglassful of infusion or decoction three times a day.

### Feverfew (Chrysanthemum Parthenium)
Synonym: Bachelor's Buttons.
Part used: Herb.
Uses: Aperient (to facilitate bowel movement), carminative and stimulant. This is an excellent herb for relieving menstrual discomforts and to calm nervousness.
Dosage: Half a teacupful of the infusion at frequent intervals.

### Garlic (Allium sativum)
Synonym: Poor Man's Treacle.
Part used: Bulb.
Uses: Diuretic, diaphoretic, stimulant and antiseptic (agent to prevent infection). Used in cookery, it's an excellent aid to digestion.

Dosage: In the form of garlic perles, available in health food stores, check bottle label for suggested dosage. In cooking, use freely.

**Guelder Rose (Viburnum opulus)**
Synonyms: Cramp Bark, Squaw Bark, Snowball Tree and High Cranberry.
Part used: Bark.
Uses: Sedative and antispasmodic.
Dosage: A wineglassful of the decoction three times daily or when needed.

**Horehound, Black (Ballota nigra)**
Synonyms: Black Stinking Horehound and Marrubium nigrum.
Part used: Herb.
Uses: Stimulant and antispasmodic. Equally beneficial in cases of suppressed menses and in menorrhagia (excessive flow), because the herb re-establishes physiological balance.
Dosage: A wineglassful of cold infusion three times a day.

**Lady's Mantle (Alchemilla vulgaris)**
Parts used: Herb, root.
Uses: Astringent (binding; checking bleeding) and styptic (contracting blood vessels to stop bleeding). Valuable treatment in the case of excessive menstruation.
Dosage: A teacupful of the infusion or decoction as required.

**Lady's Slipper (Cypripedum pubescens)**
Synonyms: Lady's Shoe, Nerve Root, Noah's Ark and Yellow Lady's Slipper.
Part used: Root.
Uses: Sedative and antispasmodic.
Dosage: A wineglassful of cold decoction three times a day.

**Life Root (Senecio aureus)**
Synonyms: Groundsel, Golden or Squaw Weed and Golden Senecio.
Part used: Herb.
Uses: Diuretic, emmenagogue and astringent.
Dosage: ½ to 1 drachm (1.8-3.6ml) of the fluid extract.

**Motherwort (Leonurus cardiaca)**
Part used: Herb.
Uses: Emmenagogue, diaphoretic, antispasmodic, nervine (to calm the nerves) and tonic.
Dosage: A wineglassful of the infusion when required.

**Mugwort (Artemisia vulgaris)**
Synonym: Felon Herb.
Parts used: Leaves and flowers.
Uses: Relaxant and emmenagogue. Helps to regulate the periods and to relieve spasms.
Dosage: A wineglassful of the infusion three times a day.

**Parsley (Carum petroselinum)**
Parts used: Roots, seeds, leaves.
Uses: Tonic, carminative, aperient and especially for diuretic properties. Particularly helpful in suppressed and painful menstruation.
   Parsley is very rich in vitamins A and C. It also contains calcium and phosphorus. Use it liberally in cooking.
Dosage: A cupful of the tea, as required.

**Pennyroyal (Mentha Pulegium)**
Part used: Herb.
Uses: Antispasmodic, carminative, diaphoretic and stimulant.
Dosage: A teacupful of infusion as required.

**Peppermint (Mentha piperita)**
Synonym: Brandy Mint.

Part used: Herb.
Uses: Antispasmodic, stimulant, carminative and analgesic (to relieve pain).
Dosage: A wineglassful of infusion as required.

## Raspberry (Rubus Idaeus)
Synonyms: Hindleberry, Gentler Berry.
Parts used: Leaves, fruit.
Uses: To remedy suppressed menses and to ease various menstrual discomforts.
Dosage: A cupful of the infusion as needed.

## Rosemary (Rosmarinus officinalis)
Synonym: Romero.
Parts used: Herb, root.
Uses: Tonic, astringent, diaphoretic, stimulant, carminative. Helps to regulate the menses and to alleviate uterine pains.
Dosage: A cupful of the infusion, as often as required.

## Rue (Ruta graveolens)
Synonyms: Garden Rue, Herb of Grace, Herbygrass and Ave-grass.
Part used: Herb.
Uses: Antispasmodic. Good to help regulate the periods and useful in suppressed menses.
Dosage: A wineglassful of infusion three times daily.
*Note:* Do *not* take immediately after eating as it could induce vomiting. Do *not* take in large doses.

## Saffron (Crocus sativus)
Synonyms: Crocus, Alicante saffron, Valencia saffron, Hay saffron and Gatinais saffron.
Part used: Flower pistils.
Uses: Excellent to treat amenorrhoea (absence of menses) and dysmenorrhoea. Useful, too, in cases of menorrhagia and in regulating the menstrual flow. Also carminative and diaphoretic.

Dosage: A teaspoonful of infusion three times a day. If the fluid extract is used, take 4 or 5 drops in water every three or four hours until there is relief of symptoms.

### Sage (Salvia officinalis)
Synonym: Garden sage.
Part used: Leaves.
Uses: Stimulant, astringent, tonic and carminative. Useful in cases of amenorrhoea and in menorrhagia. Also helpful in regulating the periods.
Dosage: Take a wineglassful or half a cupful of the infusion as often as desired.

### Sarsaparilla (Smilax officinalis)
Synonyms: Jamaica sarsaparilla, Guay-quill sarsaparilla, Red sarsaparilla.
Uses: Diuretic and stimulant. Excellent for internal inflammations. Also carminative.
Dosage: Make a tea from the powdered sarsaparilla and drink a cupful daily.

### Shepherd's Purse (Capsella bursa-pastoris)
Synonyms: Lady's Purse, Mother's Heart, Shepherd's Scrip and Bourse de pasteur.
Part used: Whole plant.
Uses: Excellent for stopping haemorrhages (bleeding) of all kinds. Useful in relieving menorrhagia.
Dosage: A wineglassful of infusion three or four times a day.

### Southernwood (Artemisia abrotanum)
Part used: Herb.
Uses: Emmenagogue and antiseptic as well as tonic.
Dosage: A cupful of infusion (*not* the decoction, which is unpleasant) as required.

### Thyme, Wild (Thymus serpyllum)
Synonyms: Mother of Thyme, Serpullum, Creeping Thyme and Brotherwort.

Part used: Herb.
Uses: Diuretic, stimulant, antiseptic, antispasmodic and emmenagogue. It is also carminative.
Dosage: Take one or more tablespoonsful of infusion several times a day.

**Valerian, American (Cypripedum pubescens)**
*See* Lady's Slipper

**Yarrow (Achillea millefolium)**
Synonyms: Milfoil, Thousand-leaf, Nosebleed, Old man's pepper, Soldier's Woundwort and Knyghten.
Part used: Herb.
Uses: Astringent—helps to stem profuse menstrual bleeding. Also tonic, stimulant and diaphoretic.
Dosage: A wineglassful of infusion three times daily.

*Tisanes*
Tisanes (from the French word 'tisane') are herbal teas. Here are recipes for two tisanes with relaxing and diuretic properties.

## Diuretic Tisane
*How to make it*
1.  Mix together 28g (1 ounce) each alfalfa, camomile, comfrey leaf, dandelion, elder and lemon peel.
2.  Store this herbal mixture in an airtight container, in a cool, dark place.
3.  When needed, pour 500ml (2 cups) boiling water over 30ml (2 tablespoons) of the mixed herbs. Let it infuse for about 20 minutes before using.

## Soothing Tisane
*How to make it*
1.  Mix together 28g (1 ounce) each camomile, cowslip, linden and violet flowers.

2.   Store the herbal mixture in an airtight container, in a cool, dark place.

3.   When ready to use it, pour 500ml (2 cups) boiling water over 30ml (2 tablespoons) of the mixed herbs and infuse for about 20 minutes.

Linden is a mild sedative. Violet flowers contain salicylic acid (a pain reliever) and vitamins A and C.

# CHAPTER 9

# Wonderful Evening Primrose Oil

From the tiny seeds of an unprepossessing little plant comes an oil that promises to be even more medicinally outstanding than digitalis (from the foxglove), quinine (from cinchona bark) or reserpine (from rauwolfia). That plant is the evening primrose, botanically known as *Oenothera biennis* (from Greek *oinis,* wine and *thera*, a hunt). Its active ingredient was thought to counteract the effects of wine, as the origin of the name suggests.

## Description
The flowers of the evening primrose are generally a bright yellow colour with a delicate fragrance. They usually open between six and seven o'clock in the evening—hence their name.

Some plants grow no higher than dandelions. Others shoot up to a height of 2.4 metres (about 8 feet).

The seeds, which are as minute as mustard seeds, have to be harvested by hand. This understandably makes the end product—the oil—somewhat expensive.

## History
For over 500 years, the leaves and bark of the evening primrose were used by North American Indians for the treatment of a variety of illnesses, notably skin disorders, breathing problems, gastrointestinal complaints and pelvic congestion in females. Today, the roots are eaten in some countries, in spring, and the French often add it to salads as a garnish.

The evening primrose probably originated in Central or South America and now flourishes along the eastern seaboard of the United States of America and Canada. It has also spread across the world and can be found on every continent. It grows profusely along river banks and other sandy places in Western Europe. It is also cultivated in English gardens, and is fully naturalized in Lancashire and a few other counties in England.

For a time, in Europe, the evening primrose enjoyed notoriety when it became known as 'King's Cure All', because of its usefulness in relieving a seemingly endless variety of ills, including those of the sovereign himself. It then took a back seat to other remedies until the twentieth century.

At this time, a German scientist named Unger discovered that the seeds of the plant contained fifteen per cent oil, extractable as light petroleum. Subsequently, two other scientists analysed the oil and found that, in addition to oleic and linoleic acids, it contained another, rare, essential fatty acid (EFA), to which they gave the name *gamma-linolenic acid* (GLA).

Two decades later, a British biochemist, Dr J. P. Ripley, repeated the analyses using modern techniques. He found that evening primrose oil did indeed contain GLA.

In the 1960s, British scientists decided to investigate the oil for possible applications in the health field. The object of their first experiments was to compare the biological activity of linoleic acid (first mentioned in Chapter 5) with that of GLA.

Laboratory rats were put on a diet deficient in essential fatty acids (EFAs). In a few weeks, they lost hair and developed skin problems. The animals were then divided into two groups. One was fed the not uncommonly-found linoleic acid; the other GLA. The results were astonishing. The rats in the GLA group recovered more rapidly and apparently utilized the added nutrient more efficiently than those in the other group.

In a subsequent experiment, one group of rabbits was fed a diet high in animal (saturated) fats, while a control group was given a normal diet. The group on the high-fat diet was then given GLA, extracted from the evening primrose. The results of this test indicated that GLA could satisfactorily control blood cholesterol levels.

The brain behind much of the research on evening primrose oil in the 1960s was the biochemist, John Williams. He went on to open his own company, Bio Oil Research Ltd, where capsules of evening primrose oil, under the brand name *Naudicelle*, were manufactured.

In the 1970s, other scientists enthusiastically pursued the possibilities of this amazing oil. They continued experimenting with it and found that GLA was ten times more biologically effective than linoleic acid.

Now research on evening primrose oil has reached international proportions, and over one hundred clinical trials in thirteen countries are either in progress or completed.

Among the most ardent researchers is David Horrobin, M.D., Ph.D., formerly a neurophysiologist at Guy's Hospital, London. He did impressive research on the role of Prostaglandin E1 (PGE1) in schizophrenia. Now, he has begun to consider its possibilities in the treatment of other disorders.

At this point, it seems appropriate to ask how something used to treat a 'mental illness' such as schizophrenia could be effective in the therapy of, say, PMS. The connection seems to be that the mechanism involved in a number of disorders (e.g. benign breast disease, blood vessel problems, brittle nails, PMS) appears to be similar. What evening primrose oil appears to do is that, once it's in the body, it converts to PGE1. In other words, it's a *precursor*, or forerunner, of PGE1.

## More on prostaglandins

In Chapter 2, I explained briefly what prostaglandins

were. I also mentioned that some doctors were employing prostaglandin-inhibiting agents (e.g. aspirin) to block the action of prostaglandins, which seem implicated in PMS. These are the 'bad' prostaglandins.

There are, however, 'good' prostaglandins, and PGE1 is one of them—in fact, it may be considered the 'superprostaglandin'.

### Role of PGE1
Here is a partial listing of the apparent action of PGE1. It:
— dilates (widens) blood vessels, thus improving blood flow;
— lowers high blood-pressure to within normal limits;
— helps prevent cholesterol build-up;
— inhibits thrombosis (blood clots);
— counteracts inflammations;
— helps to regulate brain function;
— discourages abnormal cell proliferation (rapid increase); and
— regulates the immune system (body's defence against disease).

PGE1 is derived from GLA, which is the active ingredient in evening primrose oil.

### Efamol
Convinced of the potential of evening primrose oil as a unique source of PGE1 (human milk is the only other known source), Dr Horrobin persuaded a director of Agricultural Holdings to set up another company to produce and market this oil. Thus Efamol Ltd was founded, and its now well-known product *Efamol* introduced. Dr Horrobin is the UK Medical Director as well as Research Director of Efamol Research Institute in Nova Scotia, Canada.

*Efamol* is available in clear gelatin capsules, each containing 0.5ml evening primrose oil.

**More on EFAs**

Essential fatty acids, or EFAs, are biologically active components of the polyunsaturates. They are actually closer to being proteins or vitamins than to being fats. In fact, they are sometimes referred to as vitamin F (see Chapter 5, page 71).

They are called 'essential' because the body must have them to function properly, and since it cannot synthesize them, it depends on food sources to provide them.

*What are the main EFAs?*

There are two series of EFAs. Linoleic acid is the parent compound of the n6 series. Alpha-linolenic acid is the parent compound of the n3 series. Acids from the two series are not interchangeable, and the two series are desaturated and elongated by the same enzymes.

*What do the EFAs do?*

The multitude of defects produced by EFA deficiency relate to two fundamental biochemical roles of the EFAs. They are:

1. The EFAs are vital components of the structure of all membranes within the body. (A membrane is a thin, soft, pliable layer of tissue lining a cavity or tube, covering an organ or structure or separating one part from another.) A deficiency of EFAs, therefore, generates changes in the behaviour of all membranes.

2. The EFAs are the precursors, or forerunners, of prostaglandins. They are needed for conversion to prostaglandins.

Prostaglandins are vital short term regulators that contribute to the function of every organ in the body. There are three main series of prostaglandins:

— the first series is formed from DGLA;

— the second series is formed from arachidonic acid;

— the third series is formed from eicosapentaenoic acid.

## Food sources of the EFAs

Linoleic acid is the most abundant EFA. Vegetable oils, legumes and organ meats are relatively rich sources.

Gamma-linolenic acid (GLA) is found in only two known places: human milk and evening primrose oil.

Dihomo-gamma-linolenic acid (DGLA) is found in small amounts in human milk. Arachidonic acid is found in some seaweeds, some dairy products and in meat. Alpha-linolenic acid is found in linseed oil and dark green vegetables. Eicosapentaenoic acid is found in oils from marine fish.

## EFA deficiency

Of the large number of abnormalities that can occur if the diet is deficient of EFAs, these are the chief:
— Abnormalities of the heart and blood circulation.
— Skin disorders.
— Poor immunity to disease.
— Inadequate healing of wounds.
— Inability to reproduce.
— Inflammatory conditions.
— Brain dysfunction, leading to abnormal behaviour.
— Defective water balance.

Since food sources of linoleic acid are so readily available one may well ask, 'How is it possible to go short of EFAs?' The answer is that you may ingest adequate amounts of a nutrient and still be deficient of it. This is because the nutrient may not be properly absorbed, and therefore not available to tissues, on account of some metabolic or other obstacle.

## The Metabolic Course

In her book entitled *Evening Primrose Oil*, Judy Graham likens the metabolic pathway from linoleic acid to an obstacle race with lots of hurdles between start and finish. She points out that in many persons, especially those suffering from various disorders (e.g. PMS), the obstacles along the metabolic route are so great that the journey never gets finished.

Linoleic acid, she further notes, has no biological activity on its own. For it to be useful, it must be converted to the biologically active substance GLA.

If the metabolic 'run' is clear, the pathway may go something like this:

| | | |
|---|---|---|
| From | linoleic acid | (stage 1) |
| to | gamma-linolenic acid (GLA) | (stage 2) |
| to | dihomo-gamma-linolenic acid (DGLA) | (stage 3) |
| to | prostaglandin E1 (PGE1) | (stage 4) |

## Enzymes

Enzymes are catalysts, or helpers that convert one biochemical substance to another. One enzyme, known as delta-6-desaturase (D6D) seems to be at fault in some cases where conversion from linoleic acid to PGE1 is unsuccessful. Normally, D6D takes linoleic acid, the main polyunsaturate in the diet, and converts it to GLA. The GLA is then converted to DGLA, from which first series prostaglandins are formed, as mentioned earlier. DGLA can further be converted to arachidonic acid from which second series prostaglandins are produced.

GLA, DGLA, arachidonic acid and the first and second series prostaglandins all play vital roles in the body. If the first step in the formation of these vital substances from food—the D6D—is defective, a wide range of disorders can be expected.

## Obstacles

Apart from defective or deficient D6D, there may be other obstacles on the metabolic course to prevent successful conversion from one stage to the next. These are known as 'blocking agents', and their favourite site appears to be between stages one and two, between linoleic acid and GLA.

Among the most infamous blocking agents are:
— foods rich in saturated (animal) fats;

— foods high in cholesterol;
— foods abundant in trans fatty acids (e.g. processed and hydrogenated fats, biscuits, pastries, sweets and French fries);
— moderate to high alcohol intake;
— zinc, magnesium and possibly pyridoxine deficiencies;
— diabetes mellitus;
— ageing, especially of the reproductive system; and
— viral infections, radiation and cancer.

So, although you may be eating adequately of foods rich, or moderately rich, in the EFAs, your body may not be utilizing them properly. This is not surprising in view of the proliferation of highly processed foods being consumed by large segments of populations in affluent countries like ours.

### Friendly helpers
On the metabolic pathway from linoleic acid to PGE1, the EFAs need certain enzymes, vitamins and minerals to help them along. Scientists call these friendly helpers 'co-factors'. Notable among these are the B-complex vitamins, especially biotin, vitamins $B_3$ (niacin) and $B_6$ (pyridoxine), vitamin C, magnesium and zinc. A significant deficiency of any of these can mean real trouble.

### More on vitamin $B_6$ (pyridoxine)
As a co-factor along the metabolic pathway from linoleic acid to PGE1, vitamin $B_6$ is most useful.

This nutrient has helped many PMS sufferers, including those in a study done at St Thomas' Hospital, London (more on this to follow). These women took evening primrose oil in the form of *Efamol* capsules, along with vitamin $B_6$ and other co-factors, as contained in a compound called *Effavite*. This latter product, available in health food stores, potentiates evening primrose oil, thereby enhancing its action. It comes in tablet form and contains four nutrients: ascorbic acid (vitamin C), niacin, pyridoxine and zinc.

## Gamma-linolenic acid (GLA)

Whereas the other EFAs need to pass through four stages on the metabolic course before reaching the PGE1 destination, evening primrose oil (as a unique source of EFAs) does not. Since its active ingredient is GLA, it starts the metabolic run not at stage one, but at stage two instead. It therefore never encounters the obstacles, or blocking agents, which are not infrequently present between stages one and two.

It bears repeating that evening primrose oil is outstanding in that it is the only known non-toxic substance, apart from human milk, that contains GLA. (Three capsules of *Efamol* contain as much GLA as one litre—or one and three-quarter pints—of human milk.)

*Note well:* to prevent oxidation of evening primrose oil in the body, it is recommended that it be taken with vitamin E, which is an anti-oxidant.

## PMS and Evening Primrose Oil

With publication of research findings on evening primrose oil and its success in treating PMS, the oil is fast gaining advantage over synthetic hormones and other medications, some of which just haven't worked for a great many people, and all of which can produce adverse reactions.

In 1981, one of the major PMS clinics in England—indeed in the world—St Thomas' Hospital, London, did a study on the effectiveness of evening primrose oil in relieving PMS. Over seventy women with particularly troublesome symptoms were treated with the oil in the form of *Efamol*. These women had already tried standard treatments, to no avail. Evening primrose oil worked!

Sixty-seven per cent gained total relief and twenty-three per cent experienced partial relief of their symptoms. Fifteen per cent did not note any significant change. By any standard, this is a truly high success rate. Ninety per cent of women who had hitherto been resistant to treatment had responded favourably to *Efamol*.

Evening primrose oil seemed most effective in the relief of

*mastalgia* (breast pain, also known as *mastodynia*). It also significantly improved mood and relieved irritability, anxiety, headaches and fluid retention.

One aspect that appealed to Dr Michael Brush, the biochemist doing this study, was that evening primrose oil was a natural product that produced no adverse effects, as did medications in current use for treating PMS. It is therefore in accord with the highly successful nutritional approaches which are bringing dramatic relief to countless PMS sufferers.

At the Universities of Wales and Dundee, a carefully controlled clinical study was done on one hundred women with mastalgia. They were treated with *Efamol*. Their relief was substantial.

## Dosage

In most cases, the initial dose of evening primrose oil was two 500mg (milligram) capsules twice a day after food, from about three days before the symptoms were anticipated until menstruation began. A few were treated all through the menstrual cycle. In some very severe cases, three capsules were prescribed twice daily. Some women were given vitamin $B_6$ as well, or the mineral-vitamin compound *Effavite*.

According to Dr Caroline Shreeve, author of *The Premenstrual Syndrome*, recent studies suggest that the best way to use *Efamol* for PMS is to take two 500mg capsules, along with *Effavite*, three times daily, *after food*, throughout the menstrual cycle, for two months.

After two months on this regimen, the dosage is reduced to one capsule two or three times a day (after food). Extra vitamin $B_6$ may be taken in a dose of 50mg twice a day during the fortnight prior to the expected start of the menstrual flow.

## Side-effects

The only untoward effects reported in these studies were

minor skin blemishes (three patients) and a 'damping down' of mood (three patients). These side-effects are negligible when one considers the potential toxicity of medications now in use to treat PMS and dysmenorrhoea. They seem a small price to pay for the debilitating symptoms experienced every month. Another reaction reported from the use of evening primrose oil is softening of the stool, without an increase in frequency. Many people welcome this, however.

As with any oil, some individuals experience a little nausea if the capsules are taken on an empty stomach. This is why it is important to take it after food.

In rare individuals, headache seems associated with using the oil. Mostly, though, relief from headache is reported. However, evening primrose oil should be used cautiously by those having a history of epilepsy.

## More Studies and Case Histories

1.   Ten women with menstrual abnormalities, characterized by heavy, prolonged bleeding, were treated during a fifteen-month period with *Efamol* (two 0.5ml capsules morning and evening—a total of 2ml oil per day).

In four of the women (mean age thirty-two) with IUDs (intra-uterine contraceptive devices) and regular but heavy and prolonged periods (ten to twelve days), period length was reduced (four to five days) with greatly diminished blood loss. In two of these women, stopping *Efamol* caused recurrence of the problem.

In three of the women (mean age thirty-six) with heavy, six-to-seven-day regular periods, length of flow was shortened by about two days and total blood loss reduced by one-half to one-third.

Of three women (mean age forty-nine) with very irregular periods, often lasting two to three weeks, *Efamol* seemed to have no effect on one. It did, however, restore to the other two a normal twenty-eight to thirty-day-long period with four to five days normal blood loss.

Thus, in nine out of ten women, *Efamol* had a highly

favourable effect. It reduced not only the *amount* of blood loss, but (unlike certain medications) also the *duration* of the blood flow.

2.   A twenty-six-year-old domestic manager with a six-year history of PMS suffered from ten to fourteen days before each menstrual period.

Her chief complaints were mastalgia, irritability, crying spells and poor concentration and co-ordination. Synthetic hormone treatments failed to bring her relief. Pyridoxine (75mg) twice daily at first gave promising results, but these did not last.

However, when *Efamol* (three capsules twice daily), six *Effavite* tablets and 100mg $B_6$ (pyridoxine) were given simultaneously from seven days premenstrually to the start of the period, all her symptoms disappeared.

3.   A thirty-four-year-old school secretary had been a victim of PMS for five years. Symptoms, the chief of which were mastalgia, abdominal and facial bloating, irritability and depression, had worsened following sterilization. They lasted fourteen days of a regular twenty-eight to twenty-nine-day cycle.

Tranquillizers and diuretics and vitamin $B_6$ on its own had not helped her. But when given four capsules of *Efamol* a day, with 80mg vitamin $B_6$, her mood, breast discomfort and swelling improved.

4.   A thirty-four-year-old housewife had suffered from PMS for eight years, since the birth of her first child.

Her chief complaints were mastalgia, loss of co-ordination, general bloating and mood swings, for fourteen days before the onset of menstruation. Diuretics, the synthetic hormone progesterone (suppositories) and pyridoxine (40mg) daily failed to help her.

Four capsules of *Efamol* and four tablets of *Effavite*, given daily, completely cleared up her symptoms.

5.   A forty-year-old school helper, who had attended the PMS clinic for four years, had suffered from irritability, anxiety, depression, poor co-ordination, loss of interest in

sex and some fluid retention for two weeks before each menstrual period. Treatment with a hormone failed to help her, so did an anti-depressant and vitamin $B_6$ on its own.

Two capsules of *Efamol*, twice daily, one *Effavite* tablet twice daily and 100mg vitamin $B_6$ once a day caused her symptoms to vanish.

6.  In January 1982, the magazine *Here's Health* invited readers to participate in a two-month trial to test the effectiveness of evening primrose oil, in the form of *Efamol*, in relieving the symptoms of PMS.

The results were very encouraging. Seventy-seven per cent of the participants reported less irritability, seventy-one per cent said they felt less depressed, sixty-four per cent noted a decrease in mastalgia and many women experienced less pain and bleeding during menstruation.

## An overview

In her book, Dr Shreeve remarks that an overview of the clinical trials and research into the use of *Efamol* as PMS treatment suggests that it helps nine out of ten women. This is indeed a high success rate.

Dr Shreeve's own patients who have tried *Efamol* for PMS have all experienced some amelioration of their symptoms. Ninety per cent of them have reported total relief.

## Why Evening Primrose Oil Works

The St Thomas' Hospital studies point to the probability that women with PMS are somewhat deficient of the essential fatty acids. This shortage may give rise to an excess of the hormone *prolactin*. Even women with normal prolactin levels (and most individuals with PMS seem to be in this category) may be abnormally sensitive to the hormone when the EFAs (and therefore PGE1) are deficient. Thus, an EFA deficiency can effect an apparent prolactin excess in which symptoms related to a progesterone-oestrogen imbalance appear.

Prolactin influences mood and fluid metabolism. Changes in its level can bring on symptoms similar to those of PMS.

It is believed that PGE1, derived from evening primrose oil, can beneficially influence prolactin. PGE1 also seems to have a certain 'balancing' effect on the hormone changes occurring in the second half of the menstrual cycle.

## In Summary

From all accounts, it appears that evening primrose oil is very useful in correcting a deficiency of the EFAs, which seems to be at the root of the problem of PMS. It does not merely relieve the symptoms temporarily or mask them. Moreover, being a natural food product, it can be used with complete confidence and safety.

For further information on *Efamol* and its companion product *Effavite*, you may write for a list of stockists to:

Britannia Pharmaceuticals Ltd
Lonsdale House
7-11 High Street
Reigate
Surrey.
(Tel: Reigate 22256)

or to:

Efamol Research Institute
P.O. Box 818
Kentville, Nova Scotia
Canada
B4N 4H8
(Tel: [902] 678-3001)
(Telex: 019-32199)

# CHAPTER 10

# Miscellaneous Relief Measures

The healing qualities of water have been known for centuries. The ancient Romans profited from them during their daily visits to their famous baths, and the Japanese have availed themselves for a very long time of the healthful properties of their hot springs.

Water has been successfully used to treat more disorders than perhaps any other single remedy, yet we seem to ignore it in favour of costly medications that produce adverse reactions.

Water as therapy is beneficial to at least three important body systems: nervous, circulatory and metabolic. Depending on its temperature and the duration of treatment, water can increase blood circulation to promote healing, it can act as a counter-irritant, it can stimulate or it can soothe. Moreover, there are three superb things about water: it's natural, it's usually abundant and it's not expensive as a rule.

## Baths

Baths have been used since olden times for a multitude of reasons. They have been employed as a soporific (to induce sleep), to allay muscle spasms, to relieve aches, stiffness and soreness of joints and muscles, to cleanse and refresh, to soothe itching and to stimulate the blood circulation to produce a tonic effect on the whole system.

The following baths are particularly useful in easing various discomforts associated with the menstrual cycle.

## Epsom salts bath

*How to prepare it*

Put 454g (1 pound) epsom salts into a tub of warm water and let it dissolve. Soak in it for at least fifteen minutes to relieve bodily stiffness and to relax the muscles.

## Herbal bath

*How to prepare it*

Put a handful of herbs (e.g. basil, camomile flowers, lavender, marigold petals, peppermint, red clover, rosemary, sage or spearmint) into a small bag with a drawstring. Close the bag and hang it around the taps.

As the bath fills, the warm water will dissolve the aromatic oils in the herbs and fill the bathroom with fragrance. As you soak in the tub, you'll savour a feeling of luxury which enhances your sense of well-being. Soak for at least fifteen minutes.

## A Japanese-style bath

*How to take it*

1.   Shower well.
2.   Submerge yourself up to your neck in warm water of a comfortable temperature. Soak for about fifteen minutes.
3.   Get out of the tub and gently pat yourself dry with a large, soft towel.
4.   Put on a loose fitting, lightweight garment. Lie down and practise deep relaxation (as outlined in Chapter 7, pages 129-30).

## Juniper bath

Juniper berries (Juniperus communis), used in baths, are excellent for relaxing aching muscles.

*How to prepare it*

1.   Make a decoction of the berries (see Chapter 8, page 133,

for instructions). This will extract the beneficial constituents.
2.   Strain the decoction and mix it into a warm bath. Soak
in it for at least fifteen minutes.

For best results, take a juniper bath two or three times a
week.


## Salt bath

The Ward Sister of a gynaecology ward in a hospital where I
once worked, would order a daily salt bath for some of her
patients after they had had surgery. She believed that it
promoted the healing of incisions and helped to prevent
infection. She was apparently right. Certainly, the women
always looked forward to their daily healing bath and
invariably came out of the tub feeling beautifully cleansed
and invigorated.

*How to prepare it*

Put 1 cup ordinary table salt (or sea salt if you have it) into a
tub of warm water and let it dissolve.

Soak in it for at least fifteen minutes and benefit from its
health-promoting properties.


## Sitz bath

This ancient type of bath is excellent for relieving pain and
various discomforts. Its benefits occur:

— because of increased peripheral vasodilation (increased
blood supply to the body's extremities through widening of
blood vessels);

. — through the easing of pressure on nerve endings,
caused by stagnated blood; and

— through the relaxation of local muscles.

*How to prepare it*

Special sitz tubs are available to allow you to sit comfortably
with the hips and buttocks immersed in water. However,
you can use a large, deep basin very effectively.

Fill the basin with enough water so that when you sit in it

your pelvis is submerged. The water temperature should be between 38°C and 46°C (100°F and 115°F), and this temperature can be maintained by adding more warm water as needed.

Ideally, the feet and legs should not be in the water, that is why a basin is more desirable than a bathtub.

For maximum benefit, remain in the sitz bath for ten to twenty minutes. Keep your upper body warm to prevent chilling and consequent constriction (tightening) of blood vessels.

### Vinegar bath

Years ago, vinegar baths were prescribed for the relief of chronic rheumatism symptoms. Today, cider vinegar is added to water to soothe itching skin and relieve muscular aches. A cider vinegar bath is a boon to tired legs and feet.
*How to prepare it*
Put 1 cup (250ml) cider vinegar into the bathtub and fill it with warm water.

Soak in the tub for about fifteen minutes.

### Healing foot bath

One writer humorously described the effects of this bath, used to relieve some types of headache, as getting to the attic through the cellar door.

It works, though, because some headaches are the result of congestion—too much blood in the head. By soaking the feet in hot water, the blood vessels there dilate, or widen, and cause blood to be drawn away from the head down to the feet.

Apart from its value as a natural headache remedy the foot bath is wonderful for alleviating tiredness in the legs. In this case, it may be followed by a quick dip in cold water.
*How to prepare it*
Put enough water in a basin or bucket to cover your ankles.

The water temperature should be about 43°C (110°F).

Soak your feet for about fifteen minutes.


## Massage

Anyone who has been massaged from top to toe will tell you what a pleasurable and relaxing experience it is. I can vouch for this. Many years ago, before I became adept at the art of deep relaxation, I would occasionally ask my husband to give me an all-over massage. It was the only thing that would obliterate the intense fatigue I sometimes felt.

My husband would put a little olive oil on his hands and massage from my neck to the soles of my feet. He would—at my request—give special attention to the back of my neck, shoulders, the small of the back and behind the thighs. He would then throw a lightweight blanket over me, and with a contented sigh I would drift into oblivion. An hour or so later, I would get up feeling wonderfully refreshed and bursting with energy.

A professional masseuse who attended one of my relaxation classes once told me that a top-to-toe massage is one of the most loving things that anyone can do for his or her partner.

In some European countries, massage is an integral part of any health maintenance programme. In Japan, some hospitals employ therapists versed in the special form of massage called acupressure. In North America, many health spas have masseurs and masseuses on their staff.


### Benefits of massage

With the manual stroking, kneading and pummelling techniques of massage come improved blood circulation and through it better nourishment of tissues. These encourage a shedding of tensions and help to relieve the congestion which causes stiffness or tiredness. Because of the amazing nerve distribution throughout the body, pressure on a muscle through massage can often ease discomfort felt in seemingly unrelated areas. Does not a gentle circular stroking of the abdomen sometimes diminish the intensity of an intestinal cramp? Women in labour find that a similar technique, called *effleurage*, is a very welcome relief measure. This consists of gentle strokes, as light as the touch of a butterfly's wings, to the affected part. Is it not true, too, that often the most enjoyable part of a visit to the hairdresser is the scalp massage given during the shampoo? And if you've ever been treated, as I have, to a massage of the fingers, hands and arms as part of a professional manicure, you will know that the entire body will respond with a feeling of well-being.

Massage stimulates and enhances the flow of lymph and consequently the purification of the bloodstream. (Lymph is an alkaline fluid that has passed through the walls of the tiny blood vessels to nourish tissues.) When you massage yourself, pay special attention to areas where lymph nodes abound, that is, the neck, armpits, groins and back of the knees.

When next your feet ache, soak them in tepid water, dry them well and ask a co-operative friend to massage them. Not only will your feet feel like new, you will too.

When you sense a headache coming on, ask someone to massage your shoulders and the back of your neck. It will ease tensions accumulated in these areas and help to relieve the headache.

## Massage oils

Any unrefined vegetable oil is fine, but this fragrant mixture will give you a feeling of being pampered: 14g (½ ounce) essential oil of lavender and 14g (½ ounce) essential oil of rose. These are available at a good health food store or by post (see address on page 163).

Other oils to try are almond (sweet), avocado, safflower and sesame seed. Store these in the refrigerator to prevent rancidity. When ready to massage, warm up a little of the oil of your choice before applying it to the skin.

Essential oils may be obtained by post, by writing to:

Aroma-Therapy Supplies,
52 St Aubyns Road,
Fishersgate
Brighton
Sussex, BN4 1PE

## Orgasm

Orgasm has been described as a state of paroxysmal excitement occurring at the apex of sexual intercourse. Although I cannot personally vouch for the efficacy of orgasm as a means of relieving dysmenorrhoea or PMS, you may wish to try it yourself.

Some experts cite it as one way of relieving pelvic discomfort. The authors of *It's Your Body: A Woman's Guide to Gynecology*, for example, note that orgasm drains the pelvis and therefore promotes comfort and relaxation. Certainly, it seems one of the more pleasurable ways of obtaining relief from menstrual and premenstrual tensions and related symptoms.

# CHAPTER 11

# Recipes for a Healthier Menstrual Cycle

In countless homes today, both partners are working outside as well as inside the home. Many single persons, too, are attending to two jobs—temporarily working part time at one occupation while continuing their education to pursue their vocation of choice.

Time, then, is of the essence and there is little left for elaborate food preparation. Indeed, increasingly, there is hardly any time for food preparation as our parents and grandparents knew it. We are relying more and more on 'convenience' foods. These are convenient in terms of saving time but, unfortunately, are inconvenient to the budget and especially to the health. Many in the health professions are encountering an increase in nutrition-related disorders because people are consuming more overprocessed foods than they once did.

In Chapters 4 and 5, I pointed out that many symptoms experienced premenstrually and menstrually are related to the ingestion of highly refined foods in which important nutrients have been lost through processing. I encouraged a return to a varied selection of wholesome foods that have not been stripped of their health-giving properties. I mentioned some of these under the heading 'sources' of the various nutrients described. I also urged you to be more careful in buying, preparing and cooking (or not cooking) foods so as to conserve their nutrients.

Many good cookbooks are now available to guide you in these important principles. To start you off, however, I now offer specially selected recipes which I have chosen essentially to provide those nutrients often missing in the diets of women experiencing PMS and dysmenorrhoea. They are delicious, inexpensive and easy to prepare. I do hope you'll enjoy them as much as I have.

## The Recipes

### Banana milkshake

**Ingredients**
1 cup low-fat milk, chilled
1 tablespoon skimmed milk powder
1 small, peeled banana (ripe)
½ teaspoon honey (optional)

1.   Put the first three ingredients into an electric blender and cover it.
2.   Blend for a few seconds.
3.   Taste for sweetness, add the honey if you wish, and blend again.
4.   Pour the beverage into a tall glass. Sip it slowly.
*Nutrients provided*: The banana is a good source of pyridoxine (vitamin $B_6$) and the milk a good source of protein and calcium.

## Marinated vegetables

This recipe is best made a day before you're ready to serve it.

Marinate a variety of fresh vegetables, cut into bite-size pieces (e.g. broccoli, cauliflower, green and French beans, mushrooms, tomatoes, to name only a few) in the following marinade.

*The marinade*
Mix the following ingredients together thoroughly in a bowl of suitable size.

**Ingredients**
3 tablespoons salad oil (I generally use safflower or sunflower seed oil)
2 tablespoons apple cider vinegar
Two or three herbs of choice (e.g. basil, celery seed, crushed garlic clove, mustard, mint, parsley, savoury, tarragon) and freshly ground peppercorns.
About ½ teaspoon each will do nicely.

1.   Mix the vegetables and marinade well together and refrigerate until ready to serve, preferably overnight.
2.   When ready to serve, you may remove the vegetables from the marinade with a slotted spoon or wire skimmer and arrange them attractively on a platter, or you may serve the vegetables with the marinade.

Marinated vegetables are excellent as an appetizer or snack.

*Nutrients provided:* Because the vegetables are uncooked, their mineral and vitamin content is high.

Nutrients provided include vitamins A and C and the B-complex, and iron and calcium but, of course, much depends on the particular vegetables used in the recipe.

## Egg nog

**Ingredients**
1 cup low-fat milk, chilled
1 tablespoon skimmed milk powder
Yolk of 1 medium-size or large egg
A few drops of natural vanilla essence, or grated nutmeg
½ teaspoon honey (optional)

1. Put the first four ingredients into an electric blender and cover it.
2. Blend for a few seconds.
3. Taste for sweetness, add the honey if you wish and blend again.
4. Pour the beverage into a tall glass. Sip it slowly.
*Nutrients provided*: The egg yolk is a good source of iron and the milk supplies calcium.


## Fruit and yogurt shake

**Ingredients**
¼ cup natural low-fat yogurt
½ cup cold water
½ cup apricots, peaches, pineapple, raspberries, strawberries or other fruit (fresh or frozen but unsweetened)
½-1 teaspoon honey (optional)

1. Put the ingredients into a blender and cover it.
2. Blend for a few seconds, until smooth.
3. Pour into a tall glass. Sip it slowly.
*Nutrients provided*: Yogurt is a good source of protein and calcium. The fruit provides various minerals and vitamins—the specific ones depend on what fruit you use.

## Stir-fried vegetables and tofu

Stir frying conserves the nutrients and flavours of foods because it doesn't cook them to destruction. Instead, it produces vegetables that retain their natural colour, texture and food value.

This recipe serves 4 people.

**Ingredients**
2 tablespoons vegetable oil (I use safflower)
1 medium-size clove garlic, peeled and crushed
1 medium-size carrot, cut into matchsticks
1 small onion, sliced
1 stalk celery, sliced
½ small green pepper, sliced
2 sprigs fresh parsley, chopped
6 medium-size mushrooms, sliced
Approximately 12 ounces/340g tofu, thoroughly drained and cut in cubes
1 cup mung bean sprouts
1 tablespoon soya sauce (I use a brand that doesn't contain MSG)
2 teaspoons cornflour
Few drops of sesame seed oil, for flavouring

1.    Preheat a wok or large frying pan. When the utensil is hot, put in the oil and let it heat up.
2.    Add the crushed garlic clove to flavour the oil. Remove it with a slotted spoon or wire skimmer after about fifteen seconds and replace with the onion.
3.    Add the carrots. Cover the utensil and let the vegetables cook for two minutes.
4.    Add the rest of the vegetables, including the parsley but except the bean sprouts, and 2 tablespoons water. Stir well. Add the cubed tofu. Cover the utensil and cook for eight to ten minutes.
5.    Add the mung bean sprouts and the soya sauce. Stir and cook for a further three minutes.

6.    Sprinkle the cornflour into ½ cup water, mix well and add to the stir-fried vegetables and tofu. Sprinkle on the sesame seed oil. Cook for a further minute, turn off the heat and cover the utensil. Garnish with parsley.

7.    Serve promptly with steamed brown rice.

*Nutrients provided:* The tofu is an excellent source of quality vegetable protein. It is low in calories and in saturated fats.

The vegetables furnish a variety of minerals and vitamins. These vary according to the specific vegetables used. Other vegetables to consider using are broccoli, cabbage, cauliflower and mangetout (snow peas).

### Fruit salad
(Makes about 3 servings)

**Ingredients**
1 small can pineapple chunks (packed in its own juice)
1 medium-size banana
1 pear or apple
1 peach, wedge of melon or other fresh fruit of choice

1.    Except for the banana, it's best to chill all the fruit first. Then wash the fresh fruit (except for the banana). Dry them. Remove the stems and cores but not the skins (except the banana and melon). Seedless grapes may be cut into halves.

2.    Open the can of pineapple and empty it into a bowl. Chop the remaining fruit.

3.    Add the fruit and mix all together very well.

4.    Keep the fruit salad chilled until ready to serve it.

*Nutrients provided*: These include pyridoxine (vitamin $B_6$) and vitamins A and C, but depend on the specific fruits used.

## Granola breakfast cereal

Make this cereal ahead of time. When ready to eat it, add milk to about ½ cup of the cereal for a hearty serving.

**Ingredients**
⅔ cup liquid honey
⅓ cup vegetable oil (*not* olive oil)
6 cups rolled oats (large or medium-size flakes. *Do not* use the 'instant' type oats.)
1 cup hulled, unsalted, raw sunflower seeds
1 cup raisins

1.   Preheat the oven to 250°F/130°C (Gas mark ½).
2.   Pour the honey into a large cup containing the oil, to make one full cup of liquid altogether. Pour this mixture into a small saucepan (it will slide out easily) and warm, but *do not cook* it.
3.   Put the oats into a large basin.
4.   Pour the oil/honey mixture over the oats and mix them together thoroughly.
5.   Lightly oil a large baking sheet and evenly spread the rolled oats mixture on it.
6.   Put the baking sheet and contents into the preheated oven and let it bake for 40 minutes (set a timer). During this time, you may carefully stir the oats once or twice to ensure uniform browning.
7.   After 40 minutes, spread the sunflower seeds and raisins on top of the oats and bake for a further 10 minutes.
8.   Turn off the heat, but *do not* remove the cereal from the oven yet. Use the stored heat to cook the cereal for a further 10 minutes.
9.   Remove the finished breakfast cereal from the oven and immediately scrape it into a large basin. (If left to cool on the baking sheet, it will stick to it.)
10.   Stir the cereal two or three times as it cools.
11.   When the cereal is thoroughly cooled, store it in an airtight container.

*Nutrients provided*: The B vitamins, dietary fibre and minerals including iron.

## Muesli

1.   Into a bowl put 1 cup rolled oats and 2 cups milk. Cover and refrigerate overnight.
2.   Next morning add about ¼ cup unsweetened orange juice and any of the following, to suit your taste:
   — nuts (peanuts, chopped hazelnuts, walnuts or almonds)
   — sunflower seeds (hulled, unsalted)
   — toasted wheatgerm
   — sweetener (e.g. honey or maple syrup)

This recipe is enough for 2 persons. It makes a hearty nutritious breakfast.

*Nutrients provided*: The rolled oats are a good source of the B vitamins and dietary fibre. The orange juice contributes vitamin C, and the other ingredients—depending on your choice—provide various other vitamins as well as minerals.

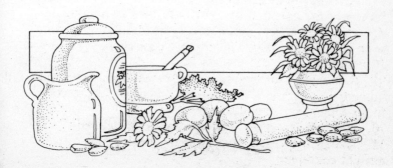

## Millet breakfast cereal

**Ingredients**
1 cup hulled millet
3 cups water
½ cup powdered milk

1.  Quickly but thoroughly rinse the millet and drain it. Put it in a saucepan with the water and powdered milk. Stir the ingredients to mix them and bring to a boil.
2.  Turn down the heat and simmer the grains for about 10 minutes, stirring occasionally.
3.  Remove the pan from the heat. Cover it and set it aside for half an hour or more.
4.  Serve it with milk, a little honey, butter, apple sauce, raisins, chopped nuts or other topping of choice.
*Nutrients provided*: Millet is an essential food item among the Hunza tribes, renowned for their good health and longevity. It provides protein, calcium, potassium, niacin, thiamin and riboflavin and has a higher iron content than any other cereal. It also provides trace minerals.

Millet is low in starches, it's easy to digest and it never produces gas.

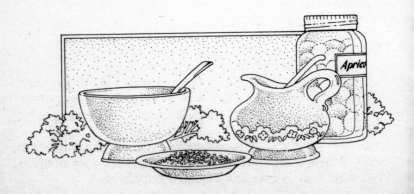

## Tossed green salad
(Serves 4)

### Ingredients
1 small bunch green leaf lettuce
1 small bunch spinach
1 large clove fresh garlic
2 or 3 fresh radishes
1 medium-size, ripe tomato
2 sprigs fresh parsley
1 cup alfalfa sprouts
4 tablespoons unrefined salad oil
Dash each of sea salt and freshly ground black pepper
2 tablespoons apple cider vinegar

1.   Wash the lettuce and spinach quickly but thoroughly under cold running water. Shake off the surplus water and wrap the greens in a clean tea towel. Leave them in the refrigerator until you're ready to make the salad.
2.   Peel and crush the garlic and rub the inside of a large salad bowl with it very well. Discard the garlic.
3.   Trim and cut up the radishes and tomato and put these into the salad bowl.
4.   Chop the parsley and add this to the salad bowl.
5.   Remove the greens from the refrigerator. Discard any bruised leaves and tough stems. Break up the remainder of the greens into bite-size pieces and add these to the other ingredients in the bowl.
6.   Add the alfalfa sprouts.
7.   Pour the oil over the contents of the salad bowl. Mix lightly but thoroughly until the greens glisten.
8.   Add the salt and pepper; add the vinegar.
9.   Toss the salad well until the seasonings are properly distributed. Cover the salad with a large plate and refrigerate it until ready to serve (for best results, though, serve immediately).
*Nutrients provided*: A tossed green salad such as this one is packed with health-giving nutrients, especially vitamins A and C as well as iron and essential fatty acids.

## Cabbage salad

(Serves 4)
All vegetables should be well chilled.

**Ingredients**
½ medium-size head of green cabbage, shredded
½ small onion, grated
2 large sprigs fresh parsley, finely chopped
1 medium-size carrot, shredded
2 tablespoons salad oil (I use safflower)
1 teaspoon Demerara sugar
Dash of freshly ground black pepper
1 tablespoon apple cider vinegar
¼-½ cup buttermilk

1.   Put the first five ingredients into a bowl.
2.   Mix together thoroughly.
3.   Add the Demerara sugar and ground black pepper. Add the vinegar and again mix well.
4.   Add the buttermilk and mix again.
5.   Cover the salad and refrigerate it until ready to serve.
*Nutrients provided*: Dietary fibre, vitamins including vitamin C and minerals including calcium.


## Nibbles and Bits

Here's a healthful snack that's useful to keep the blood sugar level within normal limits

**Ingredients**
Freshly shelled almonds, hazelnuts, peanuts, walnuts or any other combination
Raw, hulled sunflower seeds
Raisins

1.   Mix together all the ingredients. Store in an airtight container in the refrigerator.
2.   A couple of tablespoons should suffice for 1 serving.
     This snack is rich in vitamins and minerals (including trace minerals).

## Wholewheat quick-bread mix

This is an excellent 'mix' for making pancakes, waffles, muffins, biscuits and other quick-breads.

Simply take out the required amount of mix, add the liquid ingredients (e.g. milk, oil, eggs) called for by the specific recipe and cook. It's a real time-saver.

1. Into a large basin sift several cups of 100 per cent wholewheat flour. *Do not* discard the coarse particles in the sieve, they are the bran and germ of the wheat berry and very rich in nutrients. Add them to the sifted flour. Should you feel the need of additional dietary fibre, add 1 cup unprocessed wheat bran.

2. Add 1 teaspoon baking powder for each cup of flour (or flour plus bran) used. (I use a brand of baking powder that contains no alum.)

3. Thoroughly mix together the ingredients with a wooden spoon.

4. Put the mix into an airtight container, label it and refrigerate it (to prevent rancidity of the wheatgerm).

Using this mix, make the following delicious banana bread.

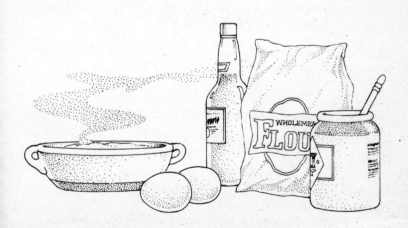

## Banana bread

### Ingredients
2 large or three medium-size ripe bananas
1/3 cup safflower oil (or other suitable oil)
2 eggs
2/3 cup unpasteurized liquid honey
Few drops of natural vanilla essence
1/2 cup raisins
2 cups wholewheat quick-bread mix (see page 175)

1. Preheat the oven to 350°F/180°C (Gas mark 4).
2. Peel the bananas and put them in a large bowl. Mash them to a pulp with a potato masher or a fork.
3. Add the oil, eggs, honey and vanilla.
4. Mix the ingredients together very well (I find a wire whisk excellent for this).
5. Add the raisins. Sift the wholewheat quick-bread mix over these. Add the particles left in the sieve. Stir well to mix together, but *do not* beat.
6. Transfer the batter to an oiled, rectangular baking pan and bake for 50 to 60 minutes.
7. Cool on a wire rack. Slice and serve (yields about 8 thick slices).

*Nutrients provided*: The B vitamins, essential fatty acids, iron and dietary fibre essentially.

## Sodium-free baking powder

Commercially-baked products are often high in salt (sodium). Since you're probably cutting down on salt, you may wish to use this sodium-free baking powder in your pancakes, muffins and other quick-breads.

The ingredients are available in chemists.

**Ingredients**
Potassium bicarbonate, 1 part
Cream of tartar, 2 parts
Cornflour or arrowroot, 2 parts

1.   Thoroughly mix the ingredients together.
2.   Sift the mixture. Repeat the sifting twice more until the finished product is powder-like.
3.   Store in an airtight container.

*Notes on the ingredients*
Potassium bicarbonate is an antacid (agent that neutralizes acidity). It is a diuretic.

Cream of tartar has mild diuretic properties as well. It's also called potassium bitartrate.

Arrowroot powder or flour is made from the root of a tropical American plant. Its mineral content is high.

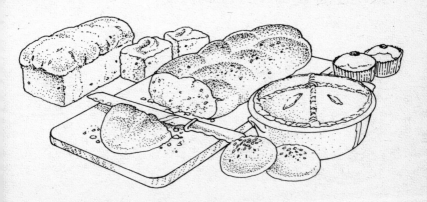

## Herb 'salt'

Here's a 'salt' that you can use liberally at the table or in soups, vegetable juices, cheese sandwiches and hors d'oeuvres:

**Ingredients**
3 parts basil
3 parts celery seed
2 parts savoury
1 part sage
2 parts thyme

Mix together thoroughly and sift all the ingredients together. Put into a shaker for easy use.

For those of you on a low-salt diet, the following herbs may be used as a salt substitute: basil, celery seed, dill, fennel, rosemary (use sparingly), savoury and thyme.

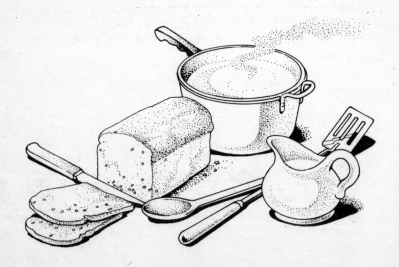

## Quick spaghetti sauce

(Serves 4)

### Ingredients

One medium-size tin tomatoes
One small tin tomato purée (paste)
1 tablespoon olive oil
2 cloves (or more) fresh garlic, peeled
3 or 4 large sprigs fresh parsley
Generous dashes of basil and marjoram, and a pinch of oregano
One medium-size onion, peeled (optional)
6 medium-size mushrooms, sliced and sautéed

1. Put all the ingredients, except the mushrooms, into an electric blender.
2. Cover the blender and blend for several seconds.
3. Pour the purée into a preheated pan, cover, and let it simmer for about twenty minutes.
4. Add the sautéed mushrooms, stir them in well and cook for a further five minutes. Serve on steamed whole grain noodles, topped with grated cheese.

*Nutrients provided*: The sauce is a good source of vitamins A and C, essential fatty acids and minerals including iodine.

If you cook it in an iron pot, it'll also provide a little dietary iron.

## Yogurt

**Ingredients**
1 tin evaporated (*not* sweetened condensed) milk
1 tin water (use empty evaporated milk tin)
3 tablespoons natural yogurt
¼ cup powdered milk

1.   Put the ingredients into an electric blender. Cover and blend for several seconds.
2.   Pour the mixture into clean jars, allowing space for the resulting froth.
3.   Set the jars in a pot of warm water maintained at a temperature of about 43°C (110°F). (I use an old electric cooker. A woman I know has used an electric pad.)
4.   Leave the yogurt for about three hours or until it acquires a custard-like consistency (until 'set'). Insert a clean knife blade into the yogurt—if it feels fairly firm, it's done.
5.   Refrigerate the yogurt immediately. I let my yogurt cool uncovered for about 15 minutes before covering the jars.
*Nutrients provided*: Apart from furnishing good quality protein and calcium, home-made yogurt helps the synthesis of B vitamins in the intestines.

# Glossary

Acid-base balance: The mechanism by which acids and alkalies are kept in balance.

Adrenal glands: Two endocrine glands located on top of each kidney.

Adrenalin (epinephrine): A hormone secreted by the medullae (middle part) of the adrenal glands.

Amenorrhoea: Absence or suppression of menstruation.

Anaemia: Deficiency in quantity or quality of red blood cells.

Analgesic: A remedy that relieves pain.

Androgens: Substances producing or stimulating male characteristics (e.g. male sex hormones).

Antacid: A substance neutralizing acid.

Antagonist: That which counteracts the action of something else.

Antiseptic: Preventing infection.

Antispasmodic: Preventing spasm.

Aperient: An agent that produces bowel action. A mild laxative.

Astringent: An agent that has a constricting or binding effect.

Atherosclerosis: A 'hardening' of the arteries, in which there's an accumulation of fat-like material within the blood vessels.

Bladder: *See* Urinary bladder.

Carminative: An agent that relieves flatulence (gas).

Catalyst: An agent that helps speed up the rate of a chemical reaction.

Cervix: Neck (e.g. neck of the uterus).

Coccyx: The small bone at the base of the spinal column. The 'tail bone'.

Corpus luteum: A small yellow body which develops within a ruptured ovarian follicle. It is an endocrine structure secreting progesterone.

Decoction: A liquid preparation made by boiling vegetable substances in water.

Diaphoretic: An agent that increases perspiration.

Diuretic: An agent that increases the flow of urine.

Dysmenorrhoea: Difficult or painful menstruation.

Emmenagogue: A substance that assists or promotes the menstrual flow.

Endocrine gland: A gland whose secretion (hormone) flows directly into the bloodstream and is circulated to all parts of the body.

Endometrium: The membrane lining the uterus.

Endorphins: Morphine-like substances occurring naturally in the brain. They act as the body's natural painkillers.

Epinephrine: *See* Adrenalin.

Fallopian tubes: Two tubes connecting the uterus with the ovaries.

FSH (Follicle-stimulating hormone): A hormone secreted by the anterior (front) lobe of the pituitary gland.

Gastrointestinal: Pertains to the stomach and intestines.

Graafian follicles: Small vesicles (blisters) formed in the ovary, each containing an ovum.

Hormone: A chemical substance generated in one organ and carried by the blood to another in which it excites activity. A secretion of ductless (endocrine) glands.

Hypoglycaemia: Deficiency of sugar in the blood.

Hypophysis: *See* Pituitary gland.

Hypothalamus: Part of the brain recognized as being important in emotion.

Infusion: The process of extracting the active principles of a substance by steeping it in hot or cold water.

Innominate bone: The hip bone, composed of the ilium, ischium and pubis. Part of the pelvis.

Insulin: A hormone secreted by the pancreas, which regulates sugar metabolism.

Levator ani muscles (levatores ani): Muscles which help to form the floor of the pelvis.

LH (Luteinizing hormone): A hormone secreted by the anterior (front) lobe of the pituitary gland, which stimulates development of the corpus luteum.

Mastalgia: Pain in the breast. (Same as mastodynia.)

Menopause: The normal cessation of menstruation, usually occurring between the ages of forty-five and fifty-five.

Menorrhagia: Excessive monthly blood flow from the uterus.

Menses: The discharge from the uterus during menstruation.

Menstruation: Monthly discharge of bloody fluid from the uterus.

Mittelschmerz: Abdominal pain midway between menstrual periods.

Neurotransmitter: Chemical substances that facilitate the transmission of nerve impulses.

Noradrenalin (norepinephrine): A hormone produced by the medullae (middle part) of the adrenal glands.

Norepinephrine: *See* Noradrenalin.

Oestrogen: An endocrine secretion which stimulates the female generative organs to reproductive function.

Ovary: One of a pair of glandular organs in the female pelvis. It produces ova (eggs) and two known hormones.

Ovulation: The process of producing an ovum (egg) by the ovary.

Ovum (plural—ova): An egg. The reproductive cell of the female.

Perineal: Refers to the perineum.

Perineum: The tissues between the anus and the external genitals.

Pituitary gland (hypophysis): An endocrine gland located in the base of the brain.

Placebo: An inactive substance used to satisfy the desire for medicine.

PMS (premenstrual syndrome): A set of symptoms occurring between the middle of the menstrual cycle and the beginning of the menstrual flow.

Progesterone: A hormone of the corpus luteum which controls menstruation and pregnancy.

Progestin: Refers to a large group of synthetic drugs which have a progesterone-like effect on the uterus.

Progestogens: Hormonal substances which produce effects similar to those due to progesterone.

Prolactin: A hormone produced by the anterior (front) lobe of the pituitary gland. It has several metabolic functions.

Pubis: *See* Symphysis pubis.

Rectum: The lower end of the large intestine.

Sacro-iliac joints: The joints formed by the hip bones and the sacrum.

Sacrum: A triangular bone located above the coccyx ('tail bone'). It forms the back of the pelvis.

Symphysis pubis: The junction of the pubic bones at midline in front. The bony prominence under the pubic hair.

Syndrome: A group of symptoms typical of a particular disorder or disease.

Thyroid gland: A two-lobed endocrine gland located in front of the wind-pipe.

Thyroxine: A hormone secreted by the thyroid gland.

Urinary bladder: The reservoir for urine.

Uterine tubes: *See* Fallopian tubes.

Uterus: The womb. A triangular, hollow muscle organ located in the pelvis.

Vacuum headache: A type of headache due to the swelling of the cells at the entrance to the nasal sinuses.

Vagina: The canal leading from the neck of the uterus to the external genitals.

Vertebra (plural vertebrae): Any one of the thirty-three irregular bones making up the spinal column.

Vertebral column (spinal column or spine): The backbone, composed of thirty-three vertebrae.

# Bibliography

Airola, Paavo, Ph.D., N.D., *Dr Airola's Handbook of Natural Healing: How to Get Well* (Health Plus Publishers, 1974).
——, *Everywoman's Book* (Health Plus Publishers, 1979).
Ajemian, Ina, and Balfour M. Mount (Eds), *The R.V.H. Manual on Palliative/Hospice Care* (Arno Press, 1980).
Beckett, Sarah, *Herbs for Feminine Ailments* (Thorsons, 1973).
Boston Women's Health Book Collective, The, *Our Bodies, Our Selves* (2nd ed.) (Simon and Schuster, 1976; British edition, Penguin, 1979).
Brena, Steven, M.D., *Pain and Religion* (Charles C. Thomas, 1972).
——, *Yoga and Medicine* (Penguin Books Inc., 1973).
Bricklin, Mark, *The Practical Encyclopedia of Natural Healing* (Rodale Press Inc., 1976).
Cherry, Sheldon H., M.D., *For Women of All Ages. A Gynaecologist's Guide to Modern Female Health Care* (Macmillan Publishing Co. Inc., 1979).
Cohen-Rose, Sandra, and Dr Colin Penfield Rose, *The New Canadian High Energy Diet* (Corona Publishers, 1982).
Dalton, Katharina, M.D., *Once A Month* (Hunter House Inc., 1979).
Davis, Adelle, *Let's Eat Right to Keep Fit* (The New American Library Inc., 1970).
——, *Let's Get Well* (The New American Library of Canada Limited, 1972).
Ellis, J. M., *Vitamin $B_6$: The Doctor's Report* (Harper and Row, 1973).
Gelb, Harold, D.M.D., and Siegel, Paula M., *Killing Pain Without Prescription* (Thorsons, 1983).

Graham, Judy, *Evening Primrose Oil* (Thorsons, 1984).

Grieve, Mrs M., F.R.H.S., *A Modern Herbal* (Dover Publications, Inc., 1971).

Houck, Catherine, 'Psychosomatic Illness is Much More Than You Imagined.' *Cosmopolitan*, October, 1983, p. 292.

Hopson, Janet, and Rosenfeld, Ann, 'PMS: Puzzling Monthly Symptoms.' *Psychology Today*, August 1984, pp. 30-35.

Jacobson, Edmund, M.D., *You Must Relax* (4th ed.) (McGraw-Hill Book Company Inc., 1962).

Jones, D. Yvonne, M.S., and Shiribi K. Kumanyika, Ph.D., 'Premenstrual Syndrome: A Review of Possible Dietary Influences.' *Journal of the Canadian Dietetic Association*, Vol. 44, No. 3, July 1983.

Kinch, Robert A. H., M.D., F.R.C.S. (C), 'The Premenstrual Syndrome' *Annals RCPSC*, Vol. 15, No. 6, September 1982, pp. 469-474.

King, Eunice M., R.N., M.Ed., F.A.A.N., Lynn Wieck, R.N., M.S.N., and Marilyn Dyer, R.N., M.S.N., *Illustrated Manual of Nursing Techniques* (J. B. Lippincott Company, 1981).

Kloss, Jethro, *Back to Eden* (Beneficial Books, 1972)

Kolodzey, Jody, 'Nutrients to help uncramp your style' *Prevention*, November 1982).

Lauersen, Niels, M.D., and Steven Whitney, *It's Your Body: A Woman's Guide to Gynaecology* (Berkley Books, 1983).

Lauersen, Niels, M.D., and Eileen Stukane, *Listen to Your Body. A Gynecologist Answers Women's Most Intimate Questions* (Berkley Books, 1983).

——, *Premenstrual Syndrome and You* (Simon and Schuster, Inc., 1983).

Lazarus, R. S., *Patterns of Adjustment* (3rd ed.) (McGraw-Hill Book Company, 1976).

Lever, Judy, with Dr Michael G. Brush, *Pre-Menstrual Tension* (McGraw-Hill Book Company, 1981).

Loebl, Suzanne, and George Spratto, Ph.D., *The Nurse's Drug Handbook* (John Wiley & Sons, 1980).

Lucas, Laurie, 'The "Curse"? What Curse?' *Prevention*, October 1980, pp. 100-103.

Lucas, Richard, *Common & Uncommon Uses of Herbs for Healthful Living* (Arco Publishing Company, Inc., 1972).

Mazer, Eileen, 'There's New Help for Those Monthly Blues' *Prevention*, August 1983, pp. 49-55.

Mitchell, Pamela Holsclaw, and Anne Loustau, *Concepts Basic to Nursing* (McGraw-Hill Book Company, 1981).

Nursing 82 Books, Nursing Photobook, *Attending Ob/Gyn Patients* (International Communications, Inc.).

Pearce, Evelyn C., S.R.N., R.F.N., S.C.M., M.C.S.P. (Teacher's Certificate). *Anatomy and Physiology for Nurses* (13th ed.) (Faber and Faber Limited, 1956).

Peterson, Vicki, *The Natural Food Catalog* (Arco Publishing Company, Inc., 1978).

Rama, Swami, Rudolph Ballentine, M.D., and Alan Hymes, M.D., *Science of Breath* (The Himalayan International Institute of Yoga Science and Philosophy, 1979).

Ramsey, J. M., *Basic Pathophysiology, Modern Stress and the Disease Process* (Addison-Wesley Publishing Company, 1982).

Riven, Linda, 'Premenstrual Syndrome: A Psychological Overview' *Canadian Family Physician*, Vol. 29, October 1983, p. 1919.

Rodale Press, *The Woman's Encyclopedia of Health & Natural Healing* (Rodale Press Inc., 1981), pp. 120-128.

Rohé, Fred, *The Complete Book of Natural Foods* (Shambhala Publications Inc., 1983).

Rose, Jeanne, *The Herbal Body Book* (Grosset & Dunlap, 1976).

Schrotenboer, M.D., and Genell J. Subak-Sharpe, *Freedom from Menstrual Cramps* (Pocket Books, 1981).

Sears, W. Gordon, M.D. (Lond.), M.R.C.P. (Lond.), *Materia Medica for Nurses* (Edward Arnold Ltd, 1958).

Shangold, Mona M., M.D., 'PMS is real, but what can you do about it?' *Contemporary OB/GYN*, Vol. 19, May 1982, pp. 251-256.

Sherman, Carl, 'Partners in Health' *Prevention*, November 1979, p. 65.

Shreeve, Dr Caroline, M.D., B.S. (Lond.), L.R.C.P., M.R.C.S. (Eng.), *The Premenstrual Syndrome* (Thorsons, 1983).

Smollen, Bruce, M.D., and Brian Schulman, M.D., *Pain Control: The Bethesda Program* (Doubleday & Company Inc., 1982).

*The Star*, 'Diet tips to beat women's monthly blues' September 6, 1983.

Trac, Debora, 'Healing Your Hurts With Hot Soaks' *Prevention,* October 1984, pp. 65-70.

Tyler, Sandra L., R.N., M.S., and Gail M. Woodall, R.N., B.S., *Female Health and Gynecology Across the Lifespan* (Robert J. Brady Company, 1982).

Wade, Carlson, *Natural Hormones: The Secret of Youthful Health* (Parker Publishing Company Inc., 1972).

Weil, Andrew, M.D., *Health and Healing* (Houghton Mifflin Company, 1983).

Weller, Stella, *Easy Pregnancy with Yoga* (Thorsons, 1979).

——, *Pay Less to Eat Right* (Fforbez Publications Ltd, 1981).

Wright, Erna, *Painless Menstrual Periods* (Hart Publishing Company Inc., 1967).

Wright, Jonathan V., M.D., 'A Case of Severe Cramps' *Prevention*, June 1981, pp. 63-68.

——, 'A Case of Cervical Dysplasia' *Prevention*, July 1983, p. 62.

Yogendra, Sitadevi, Dmt., *Yoga Simplified for Women* (The Yoga Institute, 1972).

Zohman, Leonore R., M.D., Albert A. Kattus, M.D., and Donald G. Softness, *The Cardiologists' Guide to Fitness* (Simon and Schuster, 1979).

# Index